KIDNEY DISEASE DIET COOKBOOK FOR WOMEN

Nourishing Recipes and Practical Tips for Managing Kidney Health and Enhancing Your Well-Being

Kingsley Klopp

COPYRIGHT 2024
KINGSLEY KLOPP
ALL RIGHTS
RESERVED

Table of Contents

Basics of Kidney Disease Diet
- Understanding Kidney Disease in Women..................9
- How Diet Influences Kidney Health..................11
- Nutrients to Know: Protein, Sodium, Potassium, Phosphorus..................13
- The Importance of Fluid Management..................15
- Reading Food Labels..................17

Breakfast Recipes
Apple and Cinnamon Oatmeal..................19
Blueberry Muffins..................20
Rice Pudding..................21
Peachy Keen Smoothie..................22
Egg White Scramble..................23
Toast with Apple Butter..................24
Cream of Wheat..................25
Vegetable Hash..................26
Polenta Porridge..................27
Cranberry Scones..................28
Pineapple Rice Breakfast Bowl..................29
Stuffed Avocado..................30
Cherry Almond Bars..................31
Pearled Barley with Apples..................32
Zucchini Bread..................33
Cornmeal Porridge..................34
Oat Bran Muffins..................35
Pumpkin Soup..................36
Maple Syrup Granola..................37
Lemon Ricotta Pancakes..................38
Buckwheat Porridge..................39
Strawberry Smoothie..................40

Lunch Recipes
Cucumber Sandwiches..................41
Summer Rice Salad..................42
Pasta Salad..................43
Vegetable Stir-Fry..................44
Beetroot and Onion Salad..................45
Mushroom Soup..................46

Rice Paper Rolls..47
Egg Salad...48
Roasted Bell Pepper Soup..49
Pita Pockets..50
Celery Sticks with Hummus..51
Carrot Ginger Soup...52
Cauliflower Steak..53
Parsley and Lemon Pasta..54
Mixed Berry Salad...55
Garlic Mashed Potatoes..56
Vegetable Kabobs...57
Cornflake Cereal with Almond Milk..58
Poached Eggs on Baby Kale..59
Apple Cinnamon Pancakes...60
Asparagus Spears...61
Spaghetti Squash with Tomato Sauce..62

Dinner Recipes
Grilled Zucchini and Squash...63
Cabbage Stir-Fry...64
Carrot Risotto..65
Garlic Butter Baked Tilapia...66
Baked Apple and Fennel...67
Herb-Roasted Potatoes...68
Mixed Vegetable Grill..69
Cauliflower Soup...70
Egg White Frittata...71
Stuffed Tomato with Rice..72
Pasta Primavera..73
Garlic Spinach Sauté...74
Lemon Herb Pasta...75
Sautéed Mushrooms and Onions..76
Roasted Root Vegetables..77
Cucumber Gazpacho...78
Broccoli and Carrot Stir Fry..79
Spaghetti Squash with Herbs...80
Tomato and Basil Bruschetta..81
Coleslaw with Vinegar Dressing...82

Soups & Salads Recipes
Celery Soup...83
Barley Vegetable Soup..84

Leek and Potato Soup..85
Green Bean Soup..86
Turnip Soup..87
Asparagus Soup..88
Squash and Apple Soup..89
Cucumber Dill Soup..90
Parsnip Soup...91
Red Bell Pepper Soup...92
Iceberg Lettuce with Radishes...93
Shredded Beet and Carrot Salad..94
Borscht (Beet Soup)..95
Chilled Asparagus Salad...96
Roasted Bell Pepper Salad..97
Tomato and Cucumber Gazpacho Salad..98
Endive and Pear Salad..99
Jicama Salad...100
Radish and Green Onion Salad..101
Mixed Greens with Apple Slices..102

Snacks and Sides
Apple Chips..103
Rice Cakes with Unsweetened Apple Sauce..104
Homemade Popcorn...105
Cucumber and Dill Bites..106
Garlic Toast..107
Baked Parsnip Fries...108
Zucchini Chips...109
Carrot Sticks with Homemade Tzatziki...110
Puffed Rice Bars...111
Lemon Pepper Cucumbers...112
Pickled Radishes..113
Steamed Carrots with Dill...114
Mashed Turnips with Garlic..115
Sautéed Spinach with Garlic...116
Onion and Herb Stuffed Mushrooms..117
Roasted Beetroot..118
Green Bean Almondine..119
Pea and Carrot Salad...120
Oven-Roasted Leeks...121
Chilled Cucumber Soup...122

To show our appreciation for your purchase, we're delighted to offer you these special bonuses as a heartfelt thank you.

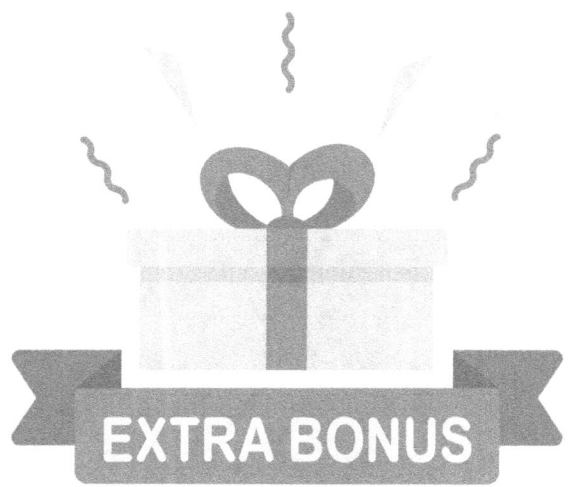

1. A Food Tracker Journal
2. Downloadable E-BOOK featuring full-color images of finished recipes

Important Note

Thank you for choosing the **Kidney Disease Diet Cookbook for Women** as your guide to navigating a kidney-friendly lifestyle. This cookbook is designed with care and consideration, offering a wide array of delicious recipes tailored to support your health journey. However, it is important to recognize that individual dietary needs can vary significantly based on personal health conditions and medical advice.

As you explore these recipes, we encourage you to adjust the ingredients and portions to suit your specific dietary requirements and preferences. The nutritional information provided is approximate and may vary depending on the exact ingredients and brands you use. This flexibility is essential to ensure that your diet remains balanced and effective in managing your kidney health.

We strongly recommend consulting with your healthcare provider or a registered dietitian before making any significant changes to your diet. They can offer personalized guidance and help you make informed decisions that best support your unique health needs. If you encounter any confusion or have questions along the way, seeking professional advice is always a wise choice.

Furthermore, If our cookbook has brought joy to your kitchen and table, we'd be thrilled to hear about your experiences in an Amazon review. On the flip side, if you stumble upon any hiccups while exploring our recipes, don't hesitate to get in touch at **kloppkingsley@gmail.com**. We're here to support your cooking journey every step of the way.

Our goal is to empower you with knowledge and culinary inspiration, but your health and safety are paramount. We hope this cookbook serves as a valuable resource on your journey to better kidney health, and we wish you all the best in your pursuit of wellness.

Introduction.

Welcome to the **Kidney Disease Diet Cookbook for Women**. If you're holding this book in your hands, you're likely on a journey that no one ever expects to take—a journey through the complexities of kidney disease. Whether you've recently been diagnosed or have been managing this condition for some time, you understand the profound impact it has on your daily life. This cookbook is designed with you in mind, providing not just recipes but a sense of hope, empowerment, and the tools to take control of your health. Kidney disease can be overwhelming, with its myriad of dietary restrictions and the constant vigilance required to maintain your health. As women, we often find ourselves juggling multiple roles and responsibilities, and adding the management of a chronic illness to that list can seem daunting. But here's the good news: with the right dietary adjustments, you can alleviate symptoms, slow the progression of the disease, and improve your overall quality of life. This book is more than just a collection of recipes. It's a testament to resilience and adaptability. It's a celebration of the power of nutrition to heal and nourish, tailored specifically for the unique needs of women with kidney disease. The recipes you'll find within these pages are crafted to be both delicious and kidney-friendly, proving that you don't have to sacrifice flavor or enjoyment in your meals.

Imagine starting your day with a soothing, nutrient-rich breakfast that sets a positive tone for the hours ahead. Picture yourself enjoying a hearty, satisfying lunch that fuels your body and keeps you energized. Envision dinners that bring comfort and joy, even as they adhere to the dietary guidelines necessary for your health. This is not a dream—it's entirely possible with the recipes and tips provided in this cookbook. We understand that every person's experience with kidney disease is unique. That's why we've included a variety of recipes that can be adjusted to meet your specific needs. Each recipe is accompanied by nutritional information to help you make informed decisions. Remember, these figures are approximate and can vary depending on the exact ingredients you use. It's important to consult with your healthcare provider or a registered dietitian to tailor these recipes to your personal dietary requirements.

As you embark on this culinary journey, know that you are not alone. Many women have walked this path and have found strength and comfort in making thoughtful, informed choices about their diets. Let this cookbook be your companion, your source of inspiration, and your guide to creating meals that support your health and bring joy to your table.

We invite you to explore, experiment, and embrace the possibilities that lie ahead. Each recipe is a step towards better health, each meal an opportunity to nourish your body and soul. Thank you for allowing us to be a part of your journey. Here's to your health, your resilience, and your unwavering spirit.

With heartfelt wishes for your well-being,

Kingsley Klopp

Basics of Kidney Disease Diet
Understanding Kidney Disease in Women

Kidney disease, often lurking in the shadows, doesn't always shout its arrival. For many women, the journey begins quietly, without alarming symptoms, making it particularly insidious and challenging to catch early. It's essential to pull back the veil on this silent affliction, especially because its impact on women has unique and far-reaching implications that deserve our full attention. Kidney disease affects the body's ability to clean blood, balance minerals, and remove excess fluids. It's a stealthy operator, often progressing slowly and going undetected until significant damage has occurred. For women, the stakes are even higher due to various physiological and socio-economic factors that can alter the disease's trajectory.

Firstly, let's talk about the unique health dynamics in women. Women undergo various physiological changes during their lifetime, such as menstruation, pregnancy, and menopause, which can influence kidney health. For instance, pregnancy-related complications like pre-eclampsia or gestational hypertension can have long-lasting effects on kidney function. These conditions stress the kidneys, and in some cases, the impact lingers long after childbirth, quietly escalating into chronic kidney disease (CKD). The symptoms of kidney disease are often vague and easily mistaken for less serious health issues, which is why they can be so deceiving. Fatigue, a seemingly everyday complaint, can be one of the earliest signs. However, it's easy to attribute tiredness to the hectic pace of modern life rather than a sign of something more sinister. Other symptoms like changes in urine output, swelling in the ankles or wrists, and persistent puffiness around the eyes are more tell-tale signs, but they often appear later, when the disease is more advanced.

Furthermore, the emotional toll of kidney disease can be profound, especially for women who often juggle multiple roles—caregivers, career professionals, mothers, partners. The stress of managing a chronic illness can exacerbate mental health struggles such as anxiety and depression. It's not just a physical battle; it's an emotional and psychological one that can feel incredibly isolating. The impact of kidney disease extends beyond individual health. It affects a woman's ability to care for her family, contribute to her community, and fulfill her professional roles. The financial implications are also significant, with the costs of treatment and potential loss of income creating a heavy burden. It's a ripple effect that touches every part of life.

Prevention and early detection are crucial. Women need to advocate for their health and insist on regular check-ups that include kidney function tests, especially if they have risk factors like diabetes, hypertension, or a family history of kidney disease. Simple blood and urine tests can help catch kidney disease in its early stages when it's most manageable. Managing kidney disease involves a multi-faceted approach. Diet plays a critical role, and adopting a kidney-friendly diet can help manage the progression of the disease. Regular exercise, maintaining a healthy weight, and quitting smoking are also vital steps. For many, managing kidney disease will involve medications to control symptoms like high blood pressure and swelling, and in more advanced cases, treatments like dialysis or even a kidney transplant may become necessary.

Finally, ongoing research and advocacy are vital. We need more awareness about the specific impacts of kidney disease on women, and increased funding for research could lead to better treatments and outcomes. Women themselves can be powerful advocates, sharing their stories and pushing for greater awareness and understanding of kidney disease. Kidney disease in women is a complex, often hidden crisis that needs more light shone on it. It's about the health of our bodies, the resilience of our minds, and the strength of our communities. Understanding this can be the first step toward better outcomes for millions of women worldwide. So, let's continue this conversation, spread awareness, and foster a community that supports and uplifts those affected. Together, we can face this challenge head-on.

How Diet Influences Kidney Health

Imagine our bodies as finely tuned machines—complex, delicate, and remarkably resilient. At the heart of this machinery, our kidneys work tirelessly, often without any signs of strain or demand for attention. These humble organs play a crucial role in filtering out toxins, balancing minerals, and managing fluids. But what happens when the fuel we put into this sophisticated system isn't quite right? Just like a high-performance engine running on low-quality fuel, poor dietary choices can significantly hinder kidney function. The link between diet and kidney health is profound yet often underestimated. Every bite and sip can impact these vital organs, either supporting their function or placing additional burdens on them. For those who've experienced kidney issues or watched a loved one navigate such challenges, the importance of diet becomes vividly clear. It's not just about maintaining kidney health; it's about nurturing and protecting it actively. Let's go into some specifics. The kidneys have a critical job: they manage the levels of various minerals and compounds in our bodies. Key among these are sodium, potassium, and phosphorus. Consuming high amounts of **sodium** (think table salt) can lead to high blood pressure, which is a leading cause of kidney damage. It's like forcing your kidneys to work overtime in a high-stress environment, which can wear them out prematurely.

Potassium is another double-edged sword. While essential for muscle function and heart health, too much potassium can accumulate in the body when the kidneys aren't working efficiently, leading to dangerous heart irregularities. Similarly, phosphorus, found in many processed foods and sodas, needs careful management. Excessive phosphorus can weaken bones and further tax the kidneys.

Protein, the building block of our tissues, also deserves attention. While necessary for health, excessive protein intake forces the kidneys to work harder, filtering out more waste products. This doesn't mean protein should be feared, but rather managed wisely, especially for those with existing kidney concerns. Now, imagine making simple, informed changes to your diet—reducing sodium intake, controlling portions of high-potassium foods, and managing protein consumption. These steps can significantly reduce the strain on your kidneys, much like easing the load on an overburdened ship. It's not about drastic deprivation but finding a balanced, sustainable way to eat.

Hydration also plays a crucial role. Water helps the kidneys clear sodium, urea, and toxins from the body. Drinking enough water is like giving your kidneys a good flush, helping them operate smoothly and efficiently. It's a simple act, but its impact on kidney health is immense. For those managing chronic kidney disease (CKD), the dietary adjustments become even more critical. The focus shifts slightly—protecting remaining kidney function and managing symptoms through diet. This tailored approach can often feel overwhelming, but it's a powerful testament to the influence of diet on our health. It's about making choices that support your kidneys, not just today, but every day. Embracing a kidney-friendly diet isn't just about avoiding harm; it's an act of self-care, a commitment to nourishing and respecting your body. It's an emotional journey as much as a physical one. There's something profoundly empowering about taking control of your health through your dietary choices. It's a form of self-respect and love, a message to your body that you're here to protect and cherish it.

Hence, how we feed our bodies can either support or strain our kidneys. This connection is a powerful reminder of the role nutrition plays in our health. As we learn more, let's foster a relationship with food that respects our kidneys and enhances our overall well-being. It's not just about eating differently; it's about thinking differently about what we eat. Let's nourish not just our bodies, but also our spirits, with every meal we choose.

Nutrients to Know: Protein, Sodium, Potassium, Phosphorus

Protein: The Building Block
Protein is often hailed as a vital nutrient, crucial for building muscles, repairing tissues, and making hormones and enzymes. It's like the bricklayer of the body's construction site. But when it comes to kidney health, the story takes a nuanced turn. While protein is indispensable, excessive amounts can burden the kidneys. Imagine a construction site where the bricklayer works non-stop without breaks; eventually, the quality of work would decline, or the worker would burn out. Similarly, when the kidneys have to constantly filter the byproducts of protein metabolism, it can lead to deterioration over time, particularly if the kidneys are already vulnerable.

For people with kidney disease, moderating protein intake isn't about avoidance but about finding the right balance. It involves choosing high-quality protein sources and sizing portions to reduce workload on the kidneys, thereby protecting their function as long as possible.

Sodium: A Double-Edged Sword
Sodium, commonly encountered as salt, is essential for fluid balance and nerve function. However, in excess, it's a prime contributor to high blood pressure, a major risk factor for kidney damage. Consuming too much sodium can be likened to overwatering a plant; just as the excess water stresses the plant and can cause it to wilt, excess sodium strains the kidneys by increasing blood pressure and swelling. Reducing sodium intake can have profound benefits, helping to manage blood pressure and decrease kidney strain. This doesn't mean meals have to be bland; rather, it's about discovering the intrinsic flavors of foods and exploring herbs and spices as delightful alternatives to salt.

Potassium: Crucial Yet Complicated
Potassium is critical for heart function and muscle contraction. It's a hero when it comes to keeping our heart beating correctly and our muscles moving smoothly. But its relationship with kidney health is complex. In kidney disease, the kidneys may not be able to remove excess potassium, leading to dangerously high levels in the blood, which can affect heart rhythm and potentially be life-threatening. The key is moderation and monitoring. For those with healthy kidneys, potassium is a friend, but for those with impaired kidney function, it's a friend that needs careful watching. The emotional weight of needing to monitor something as ubiquitous as potassium can be heavy, but understanding its impacts empowers individuals to make informed decisions about their diet.

Phosphorus: Often Overlooked

Phosphorus plays several critical roles, including maintaining bones and teeth and helping cells produce energy. Yet, it's often the overlooked nutrient in discussions about diet and health. For kidney health, however, phosphorus demands attention. Excess phosphorus can lead kidneys into a perilous journey—struggling to eliminate it, the mineral builds up in the blood, leading to bone and heart problems. Managing phosphorus intake often involves reading labels and choosing lower-phosphorus options, a task that can be as meticulous and detailed as editing a manuscript. It requires vigilance and commitment but managing it well helps maintain not just kidney health but overall vitality.

In summary, understanding these four nutrients—protein, sodium, potassium, and phosphorus—is essential, especially for those with kidney concerns. It's about more than just eating; it's about nurturing the body, respecting its limits, and protecting its functions. The emotional journey of managing these nutrients can be challenging, but it's also deeply empowering. It's a testament to the strength and resilience of those managing their intake for the sake of health. Let's embrace this knowledge, not just with our minds but with our hearts, as we make choices that foster well-being and demonstrate care for our bodies in every meal.

The Importance of Fluid Management

When we think about nourishing our bodies, we often focus on food—the flavors, textures, and nutrients that fill our plates. Yet, there's another essential component of our health that flows quietly in the background: ***fluids.*** Water and other beverages play a crucial role in our wellbeing, acting as the unsung heroes in the narrative of our health. For those with kidney issues, fluid management becomes not just a subplot but a central theme in the story of their health. Fluids are the rivers that carry life through our bodies. They transport nutrients, flush out toxins, and maintain the delicate balance of our internal environment. Every cell, every organ, relies on this aquatic lifeline. Yet, for those whose kidneys aren't functioning optimally, the management of this lifeline requires careful attention and sometimes, heartfelt adjustments. For individuals with healthy kidneys, fluid intake generally follows a simple rule: drink according to your thirst, and perhaps a bit more if you're active or live in a hot climate. The kidneys adeptly manage the excess, ensuring balance is maintained. However, when kidney function is compromised, the narrative changes dramatically. The kidneys, those diligent workers, struggle to maintain the balance of fluids, and as a result, every sip carries weight—a significance that can be felt both physically and emotionally. Imagine a garden hose with an adjustable nozzle. In a healthy system, the kidneys adjust the flow, ensuring that not too much, nor too little, water passes through, keeping the garden—our body—in bloom. But in kidney disease, the nozzle doesn't work properly. The garden can quickly become waterlogged or parched, depending on the fluid intake and kidney functionality.

This delicate balance is not just a matter of physical health; it's deeply tied to emotional wellbeing. For those managing fluid restrictions due to kidney disease, the usual freedom to drink when thirsty is curtailed. It can be a profound adjustment, one that touches on the basic human need for water. The emotional impact of watching others enjoy a simple glass of water or a cup of coffee without concern can be quietly profound, marking a shift in how one interacts with the world. Fluid management, therefore, is not just about measuring intake and output. It's about understanding the body's signals—recognizing thirst and learning the signs of fluid overload like swelling or shortness of breath. It involves staying ahead of the body's demands without overtaxing weakened kidneys. It's a balancing act performed not just daily, but with each meal, each drink, each activity.

In essence, managing fluid intake when dealing with kidney disease is a profound testament to the human spirit's resilience. It requires adaptability, patience, and courage as individuals learn to listen deeply to their bodies and respond with care. This journey, though fraught with challenges, also brings opportunities for growth and deeper self-understanding.

So, let's acknowledge the quiet yet powerful role of fluids in our health narrative. Whether managing a condition like kidney disease or simply seeking to maintain good health, let's give this aspect of our diet the attention and respect it deserves. After all, in the symphony of our health, every note matters—none more so than the subtle yet vital rhythms of our fluid intake.

Reading Food Labels

Have you ever stood in a grocery store aisle, a product in hand, squinting at the tiny print on a food label, trying to decipher what's inside? It's like holding a miniature mystery novel in your hands, where every ingredient and every number can tell a story about what you're really about to eat. Understanding this story is more than just a practice in informed shopping; it's a form of self-care and empowerment. For those managing specific health conditions, such as kidney disease, diabetes, or heart problems, reading food labels isn't just beneficial—it's essential. It becomes a critical skill, akin to learning a new language that can speak volumes about your health and help you make choices that align with your body's needs. Each label provides key insights that, when understood, can profoundly impact your well-being. Let's break it down emotionally and practically. Imagine you're on a quest to protect your heart and kidneys. You know that sodium, potassium, phosphorus, and protein are your key markers. Each food package then becomes a gatekeeper to better health. When you look at a label, you're not just seeing numbers and strange ingredient names; you're looking for clues to help you maintain your health. This can feel like a high stakes game, especially when your health depends on it.

Navigating a food label starts with the serving size. It's easy to overlook, but it's where you need to start because all the nutritional information you're about to read is based on this amount. It's like the "once upon a time" at the beginning of our story—it sets the stage for everything that follows. Next, you move on to the nutrients. This is where your detective skills really come into play. High amounts of sodium can be a red flag waving brightly if you're managing blood pressure or kidney health. Then there's potassium and phosphorus, often lurking in processed foods, less conspicuous because they're not always required on the label but just as impactful. And protein, which is crucial but needs to be balanced carefully with kidney health. But reading these labels is about more than just the numbers. It's about the narrative of health and self-care. Each choice guided by this knowledge is a step toward wellness. It's about the empowerment that comes from making informed choices, from knowing that you are actively contributing to your health with every food item you put into your shopping cart.

For anyone new to this, the task can initially feel daunting—like learning to read all over again. But with each label, with each product, you gain more confidence. You learn which brands align with your health goals, which ingredients to embrace, and which to avoid. This process can transform the grocery store from a place of confusion and anxiety into a place of power and control over your own health. And let's not forget the emotional side of this journey. There's a real sense of victory in mastering this skill, in knowing that you are taking active steps to look after yourself. It's about not being passive in the face of health challenges but rising to meet them with knowledge and determination.

In essence, reading food labels is like having a conversation with your food. It's about asking, "What are you bringing into my life?" and expecting a truthful answer. It's a fundamental part of navigating the modern food landscape, one that can lead to healthier living, one product at a time. So next time you pick up a product, take a moment to read its story, and know that you are not just reading a label—you are charting the course of your health journey.

Breakfast Recipes

1. Apple and Cinnamon Oatmeal
Ingredients:
- 1 cup rolled oats
- 2 cups water
- 1 medium apple, peeled and diced
- 1/2 teaspoon ground cinnamon
- 1 tablespoon honey (or to taste)
- 1/4 cup almond milk (optional)

Instructions:
1. In a small saucepan, bring the water to a boil.
2. Add the rolled oats and diced apple to the boiling water, then reduce the heat to a simmer.
3. Stir in the ground cinnamon and continue to simmer, stirring occasionally, for about 5-10 minutes or until the oats are fully cooked and have absorbed most of the water.
4. Remove from heat and stir in the honey. Add almond milk for a creamier texture, if desired.
5. Serve warm.

Nutrition Info Per Serving:
- Calories: 150
- Protein: 3 g
- Carbohydrates: 28 g
- Fat: 2.5 g
- Sodium: 10 mg
- Potassium: 115 mg
- Phosphorus: 69 mg

Serves: 2 **Cooking Time:** 15 minutes

2. Blueberry Muffins

Ingredients:
- 2 cups all-purpose flour
- 1 tablespoon baking powder
- 1/2 cup sugar
- 1/2 cup unsweetened applesauce
- 3/4 cup rice milk
- 1/4 cup vegetable oil
- 1 teaspoon vanilla extract
- 1 cup fresh blueberries

Instructions:
1. Preheat the oven to 375°F (190°C). Grease a muffin tin or line with muffin papers.
2. In a large bowl, whisk together flour, baking powder, and sugar.
3. In another bowl, mix the applesauce, rice milk, oil, and vanilla extract.
4. Add the wet ingredients to the dry ingredients and stir until just combined.
5. Gently fold in the blueberries.
6. Divide the batter evenly among the muffin cups, filling each about two-thirds full.
7. Bake for 20-25 minutes, or until a toothpick inserted into the center of a muffin comes out clean.
8. Let cool in the pan for 5 minutes before transferring to a wire rack to cool completely.

Nutrition Info Per Serving:
- Calories: 155
- Protein: 2 g
- Carbohydrates: 28 g
- Fat: 4 g
- Sodium: 75 mg
- Potassium: 44 mg
- Phosphorus: 56 mg

Serves: 12 muffins **Cooking Time:** 25 minutes

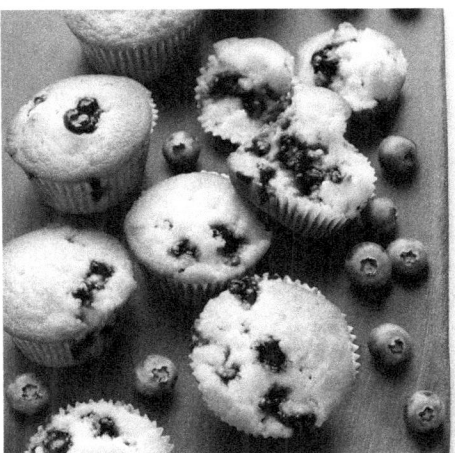

3. Rice Pudding

Ingredients:
- 1 cup cooked white rice
- 2 cups almond milk
- 1/4 cup sugar
- 1/2 teaspoon vanilla extract
- 1/4 teaspoon ground cinnamon
- 1/4 cup raisins (optional)

Instructions:
1. In a saucepan, combine the cooked rice, almond milk, and sugar. Bring to a simmer over medium heat.
2. Cook, stirring occasionally, for about 15-20 minutes or until the mixture thickens and becomes creamy.
3. Remove from heat and stir in the vanilla extract, ground cinnamon, and raisins if using.
4. Serve warm or chill in the refrigerator before serving.

Nutrition Info Per Serving:
- Calories: 190
- Protein: 2 g
- Carbohydrates: 38 g
- Fat: 2.5 g
- Sodium: 30 mg
- Potassium: 85 mg
- Phosphorus: 69 mg

Serves: 4 **Cooking Time:** 20 minutes

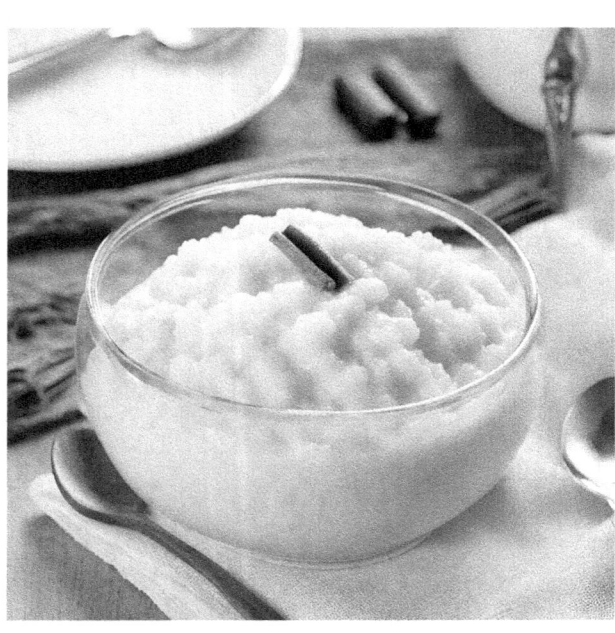

4. Peachy Keen Smoothie

Ingredients:
- 1 ripe peach, pitted and sliced
- 1/2 cup plain Greek yogurt
- 1/2 cup almond milk
- 1/2 banana
- 1/2 teaspoon vanilla extract
- 1 tablespoon honey (optional)

Instructions:
1. Place all the ingredients in a blender.
2. Blend until smooth and creamy.
3. Taste and adjust sweetness with honey if desired.
4. Pour into glasses and serve immediately.

Nutrition Info Per Serving:
- Calories: 150
- Protein: 7 g
- Carbohydrates: 25 g
- Fat: 3.5 g
- Sodium: 50 mg
- Potassium: 325 mg
- Phosphorus: 130 mg

Serves: 1 **Preparation Time:** 5 minutes

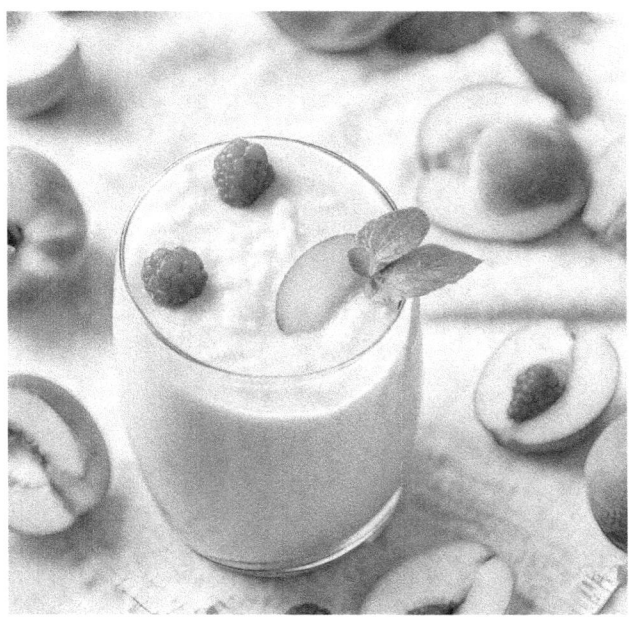

5. Egg White Scramble

Ingredients:
- 4 egg whites
- 1/4 cup diced bell peppers
- 1/4 cup diced onions
- 1/4 cup diced tomatoes
- Cooking spray

Instructions:
1. Heat a non-stick skillet over medium heat and lightly coat with cooking spray.
2. Add the diced bell peppers, onions, and tomatoes to the skillet and sauté until tender.
3. Pour in the egg whites and cook, stirring occasionally, until the eggs are set.
4. Serve hot.

Nutrition Info Per Serving:
- Calories: 70
- Protein: 13 g
- Carbohydrates: 4 g
- Fat: 0 g
- Sodium: 130 mg
- Potassium: 150 mg
- Phosphorus: 80 mg

Serves: 1 **Cooking Time:** 10 minutes

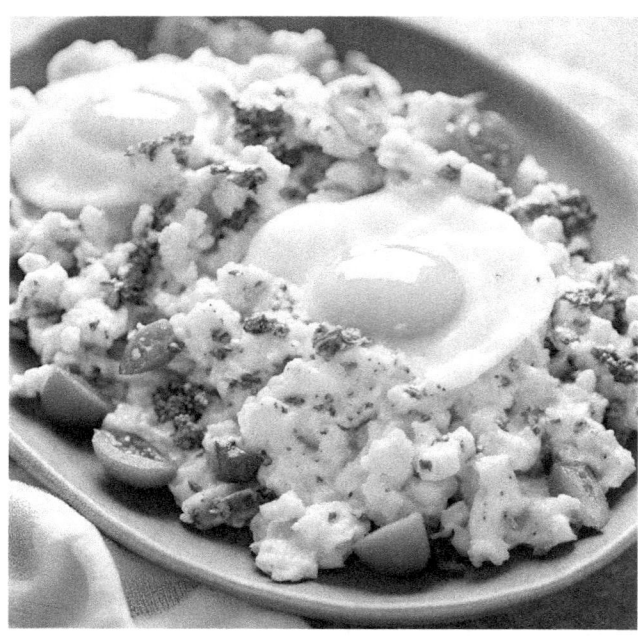

6. Toast with Apple Butter

Ingredients:
- 2 slices whole wheat bread, toasted
- 2 tablespoons apple butter (unsweetened)

Instructions:
1. Toast the slices of whole wheat bread until golden brown.
2. Spread apple butter evenly over the warm toast.
3. Serve immediately.

Nutrition Info Per Serving:
- Calories: 150
- Protein: 3 g
- Carbohydrates: 30 g
- Fat: 2 g
- Sodium: 160 mg
- Potassium: 100 mg
- Phosphorus: 80 mg

Serves: 1 **Preparation Time:** 5 minutes

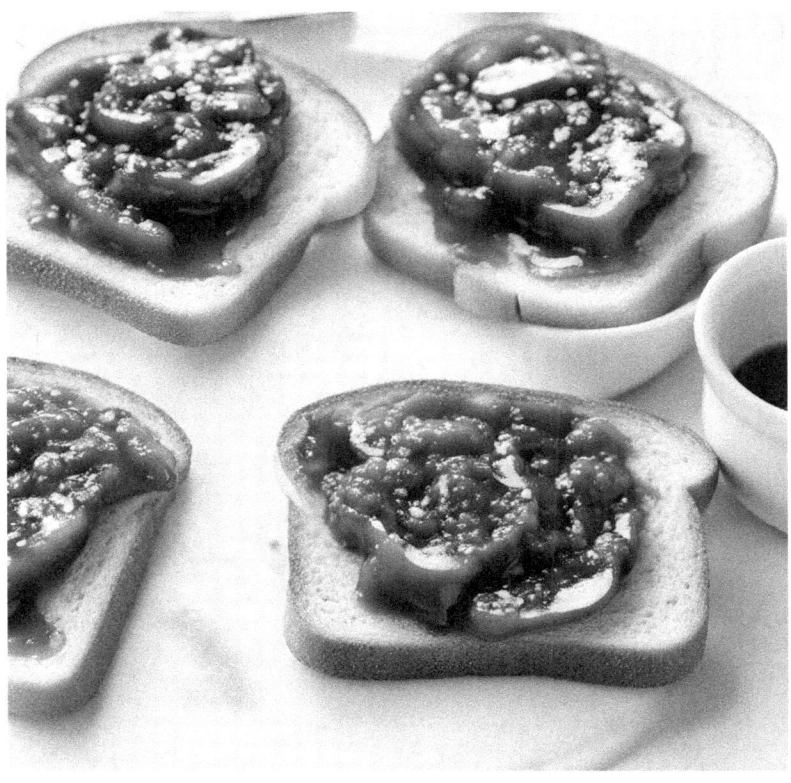

7. Cream of Wheat

Ingredients:
- 1/4 cup cream of wheat cereal
- 1 cup water or almond milk
- 1 tablespoon honey (optional)
- Fresh berries for topping (optional)

Instructions:
1. In a small saucepan, bring the water or almond milk to a boil.
2. Slowly whisk in the cream of wheat cereal.
3. Reduce heat to low and cook, stirring constantly, for about 2-3 minutes or until thickened.
4. Remove from heat and stir in honey if desired.
5. Serve hot, topped with fresh berries if desired.

Nutrition Info Per Serving:
- Calories: 100
- Protein: 3 g
- Carbohydrates: 20 g
- Fat: 1 g
- Sodium: 0 mg
- Potassium: 50 mg
- Phosphorus: 70 mg

Serves: 1 **Cooking Time:** 5 minutes

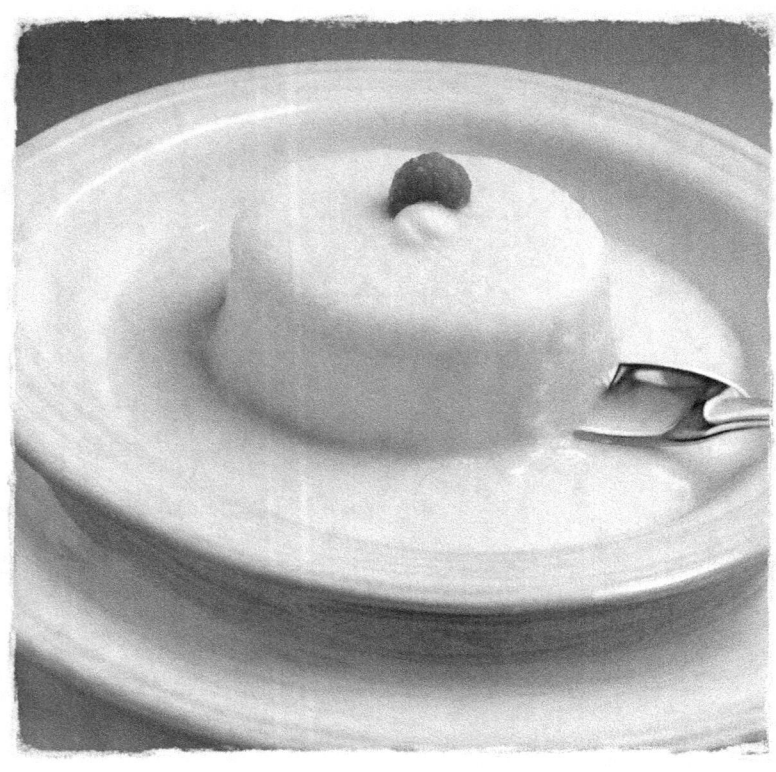

8. Vegetable Hash

Ingredients:
- 1 small potato, diced
- 1/4 cup diced bell peppers
- 1/4 cup diced onions
- 1/4 cup diced zucchini
- Cooking spray
- 1 teaspoon olive oil
- 1/4 teaspoon paprika

Instructions:
1. Heat olive oil in a skillet over medium heat and lightly coat with cooking spray.
2. Add the diced potato to the skillet and cook until lightly browned and tender.
3. Add the diced bell peppers, onions, and zucchini to the skillet and cook until vegetables are tender.
4. Sprinkle with paprika and toss to combine.
5. Serve hot.

Nutrition Info Per Serving:
- Calories: 120
- Protein: 2 g
- Carbohydrates: 20 g
- Fat: 3 g
- Sodium: 20 mg
- Potassium: 320 mg
- Phosphorus: 50 mg

Serves: 1 **Cooking Time:** 15 minutes

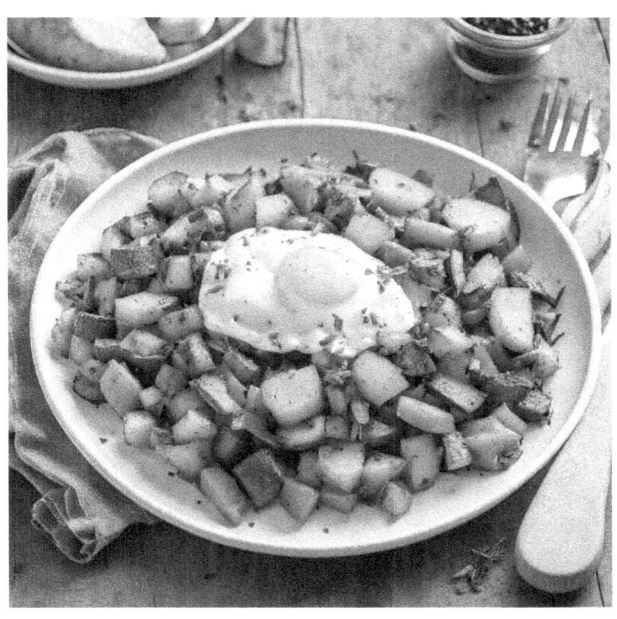

9. Polenta Porridge

Ingredients:
- 1/2 cup polenta (coarse cornmeal)
- 2 cups water
- 1 tablespoon honey
- 1/4 cup sliced almonds

Instructions:
1. In a medium saucepan, bring the water to a boil.
2. Gradually whisk in the polenta, reduce the heat to low, and cook, stirring frequently, until the mixture thickens and the polenta is tender, about 10-15 minutes.
3. Remove from heat and stir in honey.
4. Serve topped with sliced almonds.

Nutrition Info Per Serving:
- Calories: 180
- Protein: 4 g
- Carbohydrates: 30 g
- Fat: 5 g
- Sodium: 5 mg
- Potassium: 75 mg
- Phosphorus: 95 mg

Serves: 2 **Cooking Time:** 15 minutes

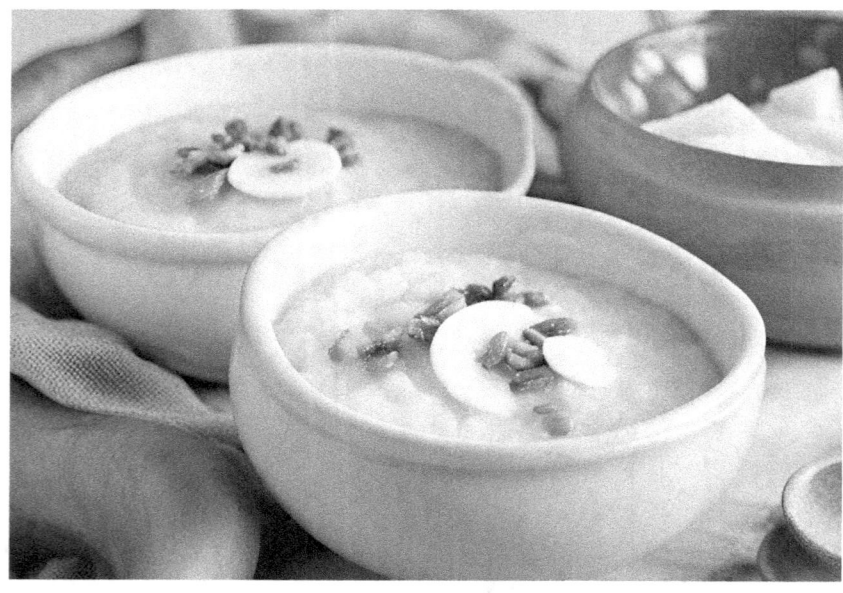

10. Cranberry Scones

Ingredients:
- 2 cups all-purpose flour
- 1 tablespoon baking powder
- 1/4 cup sugar
- 1/4 cup unsalted butter, chilled and cubed
- 1/2 cup dried cranberries
- 3/4 cup milk

Instructions:
1. Preheat the oven to 425°F (220°C). Line a baking sheet with parchment paper.
2. In a large bowl, combine the flour, baking powder, and sugar.
3. Cut in the butter until the mixture resembles coarse crumbs.
4. Stir in dried cranberries.
5. Gradually add milk, stirring until the dough comes together.
6. Turn out onto a floured surface and gently knead just until combined.
7. Pat the dough into a round shape and cut into 8 wedges.
8. Place the wedges on the prepared baking sheet and bake for 12-15 minutes or until golden brown.

Nutrition Info Per Serving:
- Calories: 220
- Protein: 4 g
- Carbohydrates: 38 g
- Fat: 6 g
- Sodium: 180 mg
- Potassium: 90 mg
- Phosphorus: 100 mg

Serves: 8 **Cooking Time:** 15 minutes

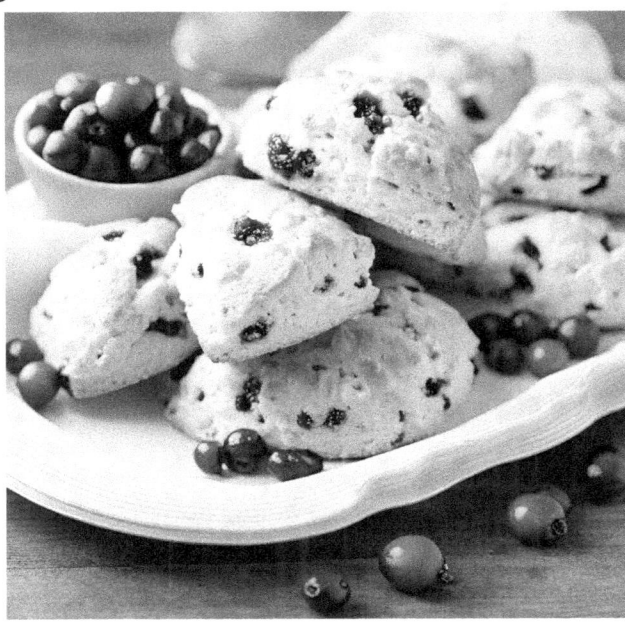

11. Pineapple Rice Breakfast Bowl

Ingredients:
- 1 cup cooked white rice
- 1/2 cup diced pineapple
- 1/4 cup coconut milk
- 1 tablespoon shredded coconut
- 1 tablespoon honey

Instructions:
1. In a bowl, combine the cooked rice, diced pineapple, and coconut milk.
2. Drizzle with honey and sprinkle with shredded coconut.
3. Serve immediately or chilled.

Nutrition Info Per Serving:
- Calories: 200
- Protein: 2 g
- Carbohydrates: 40 g
- Fat: 4 g
- Sodium: 15 mg
- Potassium: 85 mg
- Phosphorus: 50 mg

Serves: 2 **Preparation Time:** 5 minutes (assuming rice is pre-cooked)

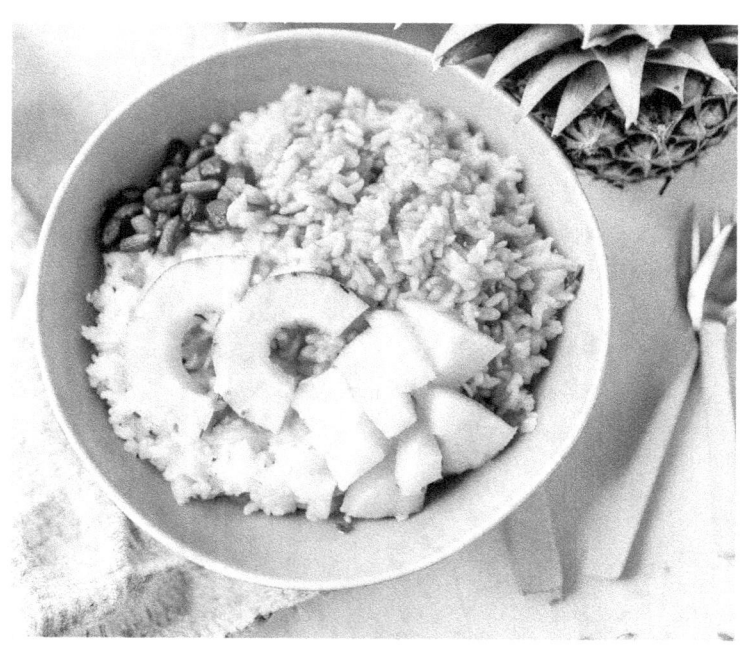

12. Stuffed Avocado

Ingredients:
- 1 ripe avocado, halved and pitted
- 1/2 cup cooked quinoa
- 1/4 cup diced tomato
- 1/4 cup diced cucumber
- 1 tablespoon lemon juice
- 1 tablespoon olive oil

Instructions:
1. Scoop out some of the avocado flesh to create a larger cavity.
2. In a small bowl, mix the cooked quinoa, diced tomato, and cucumber.
3. Dress the mixture with lemon juice and olive oil, and stir to combine.
4. Spoon the mixture into the avocado halves.
5. Serve immediately.

Nutrition Info Per Serving:
- Calories: 290
- Protein: 5 g
- Carbohydrates: 20 g
- Fat: 22 g
- Sodium: 20 mg
- Potassium: 650 mg
- Phosphorus: 120 mg

Serves: 2 **Preparation Time:** 10 minutes

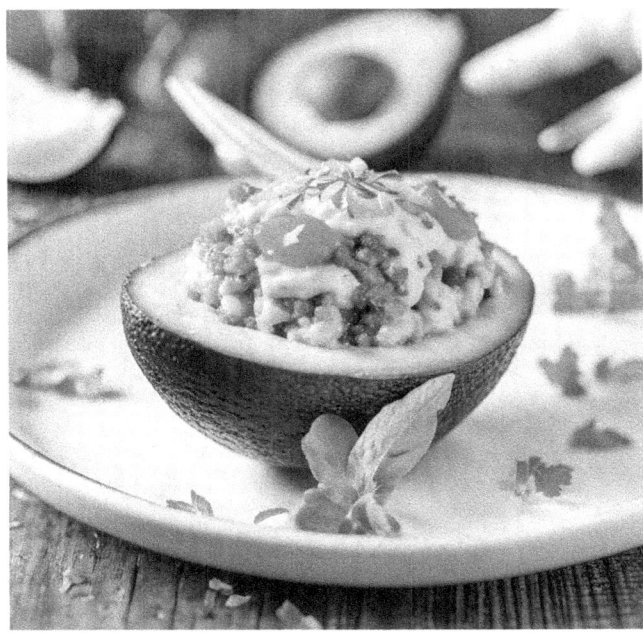

13. Cherry Almond Bars

Ingredients:
- 1 cup rolled oats
- 1/2 cup sliced almonds
- 1/2 cup dried cherries
- 1/4 cup honey
- 1/4 cup unsweetened applesauce
- 1 teaspoon vanilla extract

Instructions:
1. Preheat the oven to 350°F (175°C). Line an 8-inch square baking pan with parchment paper.
2. In a large bowl, mix together oats, almonds, and dried cherries.
3. In a separate bowl, whisk together honey, applesauce, and vanilla extract.
4. Pour the wet ingredients into the dry ingredients and stir until well combined.
5. Spread the mixture evenly in the prepared pan.
6. Bake for 20-25 minutes or until the edges are golden brown.
7. Let cool completely in the pan before cutting into bars.

Nutrition Info Per Serving:
- Calories: 150
- Protein: 3 g
- Carbohydrates: 23 g
- Fat: 5 g
- Sodium: 5 mg
- Potassium: 100 mg
- Phosphorus: 80 mg

Serves: 8 **Cooking Time:** 25 minutes

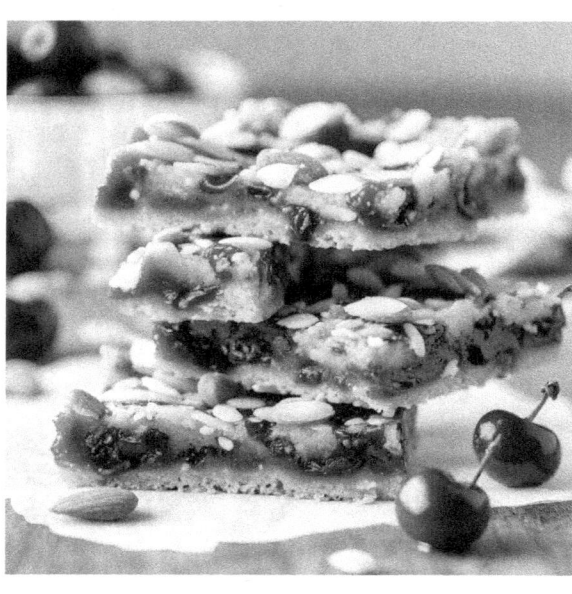

14. Pearled Barley with Apples

Ingredients:
- 1 cup pearled barley, rinsed
- 3 cups water
- 1 medium apple, diced
- 1 teaspoon cinnamon
- 1 tablespoon honey

Instructions:
1. In a medium saucepan, bring the water to a boil.
2. Add the barley and reduce the heat to a simmer. Cover and cook for 30-40 minutes, or until the barley is tender and the water is absorbed.
3. Stir in the diced apple, cinnamon, and honey. Cook for an additional 5 minutes.
4. Serve warm.

Nutrition Info Per Serving:
- Calories: 180
- Protein: 4 g
- Carbohydrates: 40 g
- Fat: 1 g
- Sodium: 10 mg
- Potassium: 150 mg
- Phosphorus: 100 mg

Serves: 4 **Cooking Time:** 45 minutes

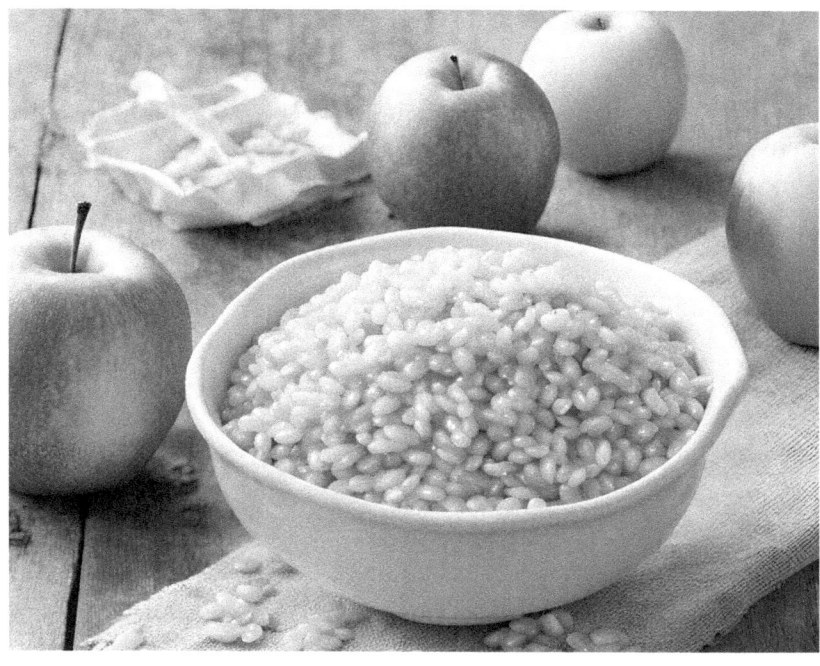

15. Zucchini Bread

Ingredients:
- 1 cup all-purpose flour
- 1/2 cup whole wheat flour
- 1/4 cup sugar
- 1 teaspoon baking powder
- 1/2 teaspoon cinnamon
- 1/2 cup unsweetened applesauce
- 1 cup grated zucchini
- 2 eggs, beaten

Instructions:
1. Preheat the oven to 350°F (175°C). Grease a 9x5 inch loaf pan.
2. In a large bowl, mix together both flours, sugar, baking powder, and cinnamon.
3. Stir in applesauce, grated zucchini, and beaten eggs until well combined.
4. Pour the batter into the prepared loaf pan.
5. Bake for 50-60 minutes or until a toothpick inserted into the center comes out clean.
6. Cool in the pan for 10 minutes, then turn out onto a wire rack to cool completely.

Nutrition Info Per Serving:
- Calories: 160
- Protein: 4 g
- Carbohydrates: 28 g
- Fat: 3 g
- Sodium: 75 mg
- Potassium: 130 mg
- Phosphorus: 90 mg

Serves: 8 **Cooking Time:** 60 minutes

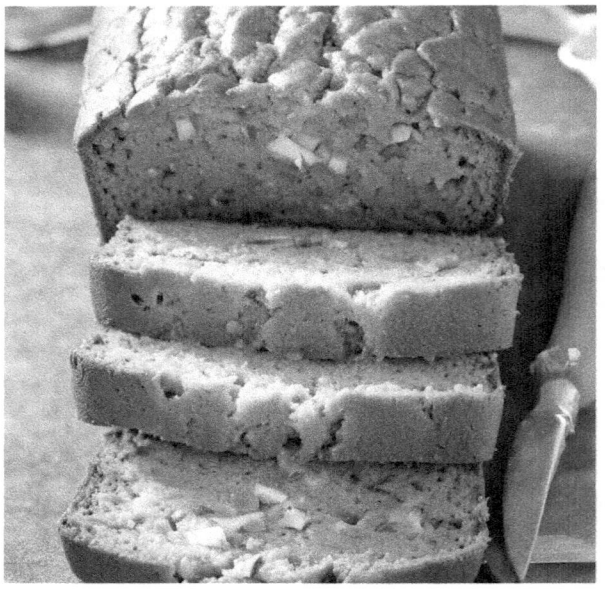

16. Cornmeal Porridge

Ingredients:
- 1/2 cup cornmeal (fine ground)
- 2 cups water
- 1/4 teaspoon cinnamon
- 1 tablespoon honey or sugar
- 1/4 cup milk (choose a low-potassium milk alternative like rice milk if needed)

Instructions:
1. In a medium saucepan, bring the water to a boil.
2. Slowly whisk in the cornmeal to avoid lumps.
3. Reduce heat to low and cook, stirring constantly, until the porridge thickens, about 10-15 minutes.
4. Stir in cinnamon and sweeten with honey or sugar.
5. Serve hot with a splash of milk.

Nutrition Info Per Serving:
- Calories: 120
- Protein: 2 g
- Carbohydrates: 25 g
- Fat: 1.5 g
- Sodium: 20 mg
- Potassium: 70 mg
- Phosphorus: 40 mg

Serves: 2
Cooking Time: 15 minutes

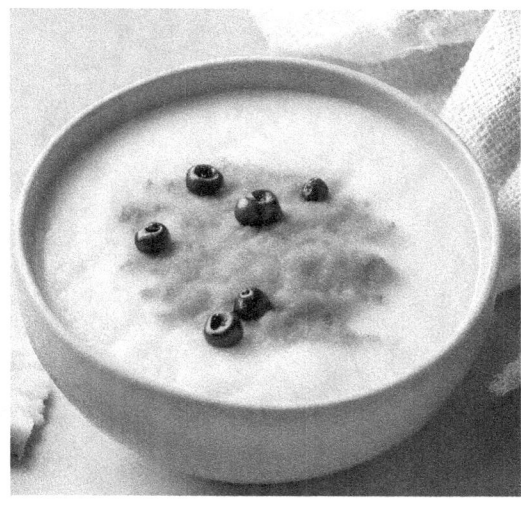

17. Oat Bran Muffins

Ingredients:
- 1 cup oat bran
- 1 cup all-purpose flour
- 1/2 cup sugar
- 2 teaspoons baking powder
- 1 cup milk
- 1/4 cup vegetable oil
- 2 eggs, beaten
- 1/2 cup raisins

Instructions:
1. Preheat the oven to 425°F (220°C). Line a muffin tin with paper liners.
2. In a large bowl, combine oat bran, flour, sugar, and baking powder.
3. In another bowl, mix together milk, oil, and beaten eggs.
4. Add the wet ingredients to the dry ingredients and mix until just combined.
5. Fold in raisins.
6. Spoon batter into prepared muffin cups, filling each about three-quarters full.
7. Bake for 15-20 minutes or until a toothpick inserted into the center of a muffin comes out clean.
8. Allow to cool for a few minutes before removing from the tin.

Nutrition Info Per Serving:
- Calories: 180
- Protein: 4 g
- Carbohydrates: 30 g
- Fat: 6 g
- Sodium: 120 mg
- Potassium: 150 mg
- Phosphorus: 120 mg

Serves: 12 muffins **Cooking Time:** 20 minutes

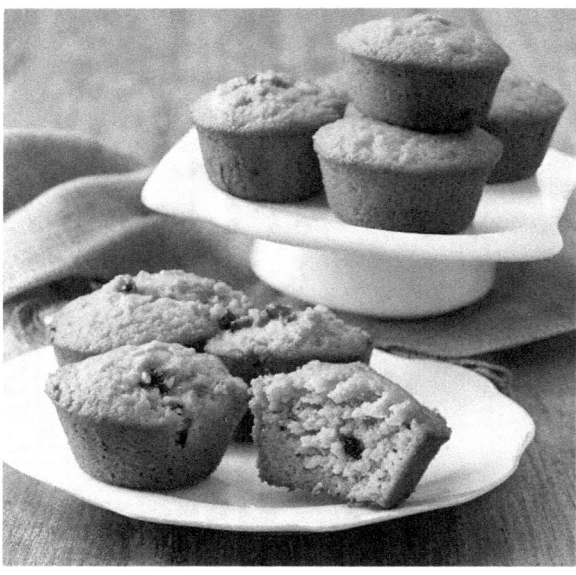

18. Pumpkin Soup

Ingredients:
- 2 cups pumpkin puree
- 1 onion, diced
- 1 garlic clove, minced
- 3 cups vegetable broth (low sodium)
- 1 teaspoon ground cinnamon
- 1/2 teaspoon ground nutmeg
- 1 cup light cream (or a low-potassium milk alternative)

Instructions:
1. In a large pot, sauté the onion and garlic until soft.
2. Add the pumpkin puree, vegetable broth, cinnamon, and nutmeg. Bring to a simmer.
3. Cook for 20 minutes, stirring occasionally.
4. Puree the soup in a blender or use an immersion blender for a smoother texture.
5. Return to the pot and stir in the cream. Heat through.
6. Serve hot.

Nutrition Info Per Serving:
- Calories: 150
- Protein: 2 g
- Carbohydrates: 18 g
- Fat: 8 g
- Sodium: 50 mg
- Potassium: 240 mg
- Phosphorus: 70 mg

Serves: 4 **Cooking Time:** 30 minutes

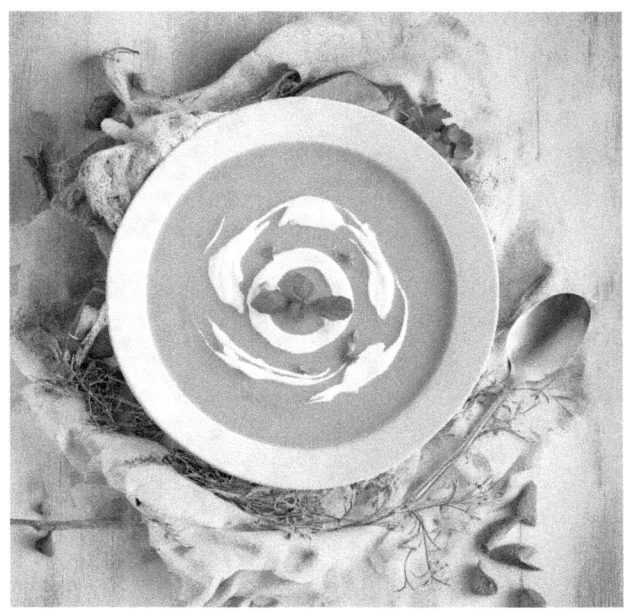

19. Maple Syrup Granola

Ingredients:
- 2 cups rolled oats
- 1/2 cup sliced almonds
- 1/4 cup sunflower seeds
- 1/4 cup pumpkin seeds
- 1/4 cup pure maple syrup
- 2 tablespoons vegetable oil
- 1/2 teaspoon vanilla extract
- 1/4 cup dried cranberries

Instructions:
1. Preheat the oven to 300°F (150°C). Line a baking sheet with parchment paper.
2. In a large bowl, mix together oats, almonds, sunflower seeds, and pumpkin seeds.
3. In a small bowl, whisk together maple syrup, oil, and vanilla extract.
4. Pour the maple syrup mixture over the oat mixture and stir until well coated.
5. Spread the granola evenly on the prepared baking sheet.
6. Bake for 30-40 minutes, stirring occasionally, until golden brown and crispy.
7. Remove from the oven and stir in dried cranberries.
8. Let the granola cool completely on the baking sheet.

Nutrition Info Per Serving:
- Calories: 210
- Protein: 5 g
- Carbohydrates: 28 g
- Fat: 10 g
- Sodium: 5 mg
- Potassium: 150 mg
- Phosphorus: 180 mg

Serves: 8 **Cooking Time:** 40 minutes

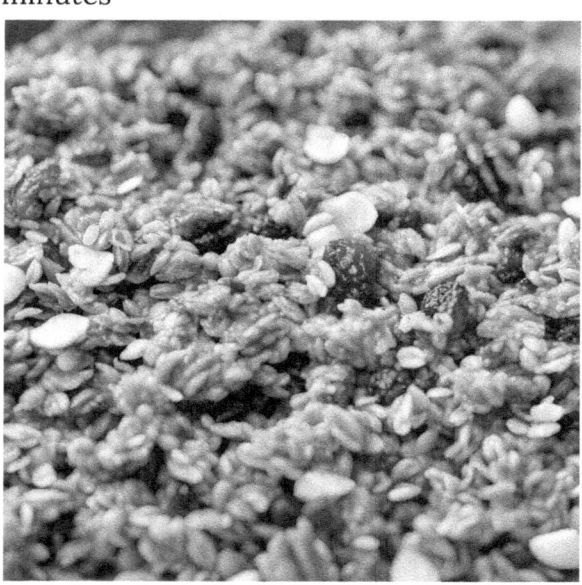

20. Lemon Ricotta Pancakes

Ingredients:
- 3/4 cup all-purpose flour
- 1 tablespoon sugar
- 1 teaspoon baking powder
- 1/2 cup ricotta cheese
- 1/2 cup milk
- 1 egg
- 1 tablespoon lemon zest
- 1 tablespoon lemon juice
- 1 teaspoon vanilla extract

Instructions:
1. In a large bowl, combine flour, sugar, and baking powder.
2. In another bowl, mix ricotta, milk, egg, lemon zest, lemon juice, and vanilla extract.
3. Add the wet ingredients to the dry ingredients and stir until just combined.
4. Heat a non-stick skillet over medium heat and lightly grease it with cooking spray or a little oil.
5. Pour 1/4 cup of batter for each pancake and cook until bubbles form on the surface, then flip and cook until golden brown on the other side.
6. Serve warm with a drizzle of maple syrup or fresh fruit.

Nutrition Info Per Serving:
- Calories: 150
- Protein: 6 g
- Carbohydrates: 18 g
- Fat: 6 g
- Sodium: 80 mg
- Potassium: 90 mg
- Phosphorus: 150 mg

Serves: 4 **Cooking Time:** 15 minutes

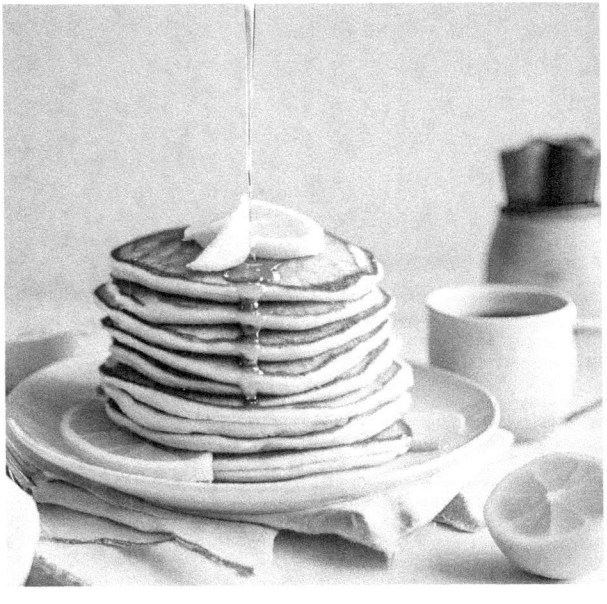

21. Buckwheat Porridge

Ingredients:
- 1 cup buckwheat groats
- 3 cups water
- 1/2 teaspoon cinnamon
- 1 apple, peeled and diced
- 1 tablespoon honey or maple syrup

Instructions:
1. Rinse the buckwheat groats under cold water until water runs clear.
2. In a saucepan, combine the buckwheat groats, water, and cinnamon.
3. Bring to a boil, then reduce heat and simmer, covered, for 20 minutes.
4. Add the diced apple and simmer for an additional 10 minutes or until the buckwheat is soft and the water is mostly absorbed.
5. Stir in honey or maple syrup before serving.

Nutrition Info Per Serving:
- Calories: 200
- Protein: 6 g
- Carbohydrates: 44 g
- Fat: 1 g
- Sodium: 5 mg
- Potassium: 170 mg
- Phosphorus: 120 mg

Serves: 4 **Cooking Time:** 30 minutes

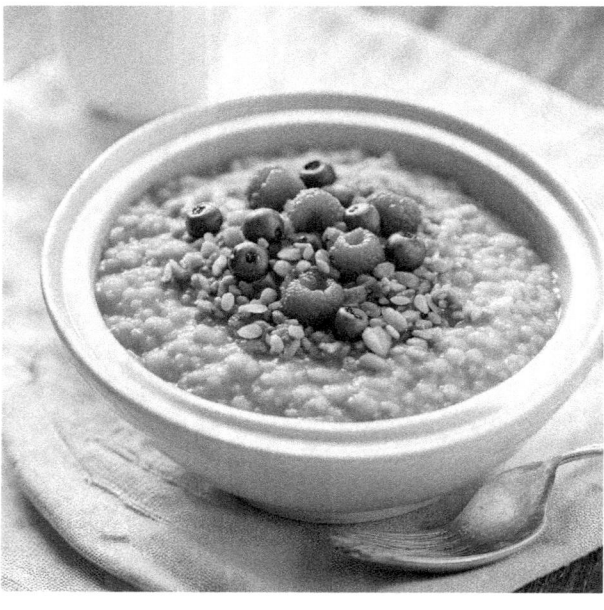

22. Strawberry Smoothie

Ingredients:
- 1 cup fresh strawberries
- 1/2 banana
- 1/2 cup Greek yogurt
- 1/2 cup almond milk
- 1 tablespoon honey

Instructions:
1. Combine all ingredients in a blender.
2. Blend until smooth.
3. Serve immediately.

Nutrition Info Per Serving:
- Calories: 140
- Protein: 5 g
- Carbohydrates: 27 g
- Fat: 2 g
- Sodium: 30 mg
- Potassium: 250 mg
- Phosphorus: 100 mg

Serves: 2 **Preparation Time:** 5 minutes

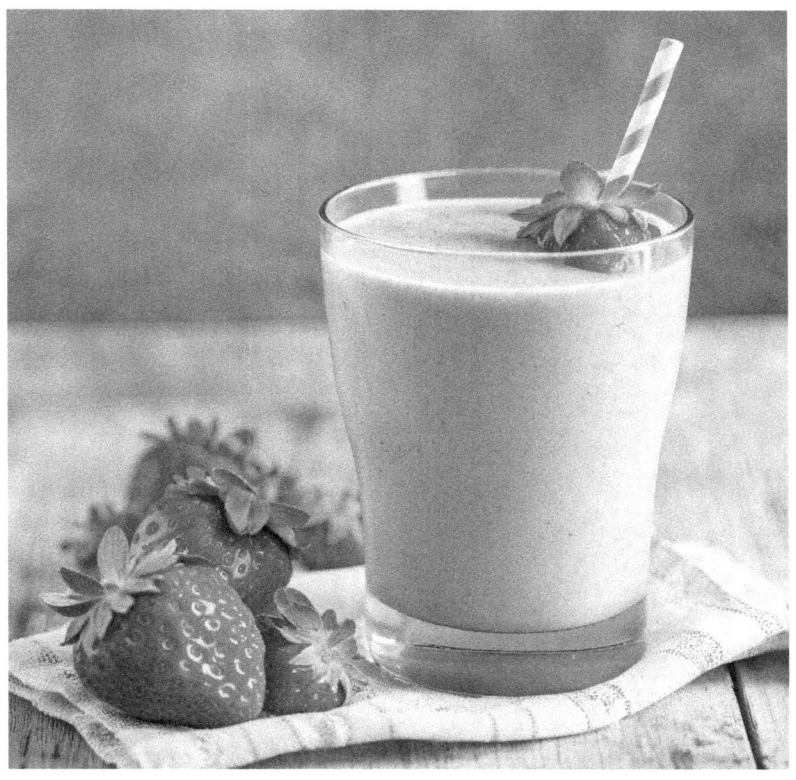

Lunch Recipes

1. Cucumber Sandwiches

Ingredients:
- 4 slices of whole wheat bread
- 1 medium cucumber, thinly sliced
- 2 tablespoons cream cheese (low fat)
- 1 tablespoon fresh dill, chopped
- 1 teaspoon lemon juice

Instructions:
1. Mix the cream cheese with lemon juice and dill in a small bowl.
2. Spread the cream cheese mixture evenly on each slice of bread.
3. Arrange the cucumber slices on two of the slices, covering the cream cheese.
4. Top with the remaining slices of bread, cream cheese side down.
5. Cut each sandwich into four triangles and serve.

Nutrition Info Per Serving:
- Calories: 150
- Protein: 6 g
- Carbohydrates: 20 g
- Fat: 5 g
- Sodium: 180 mg
- Potassium: 200 mg
- Phosphorus: 100 mg

Serves: 2 **Preparation Time:** 10 minutes

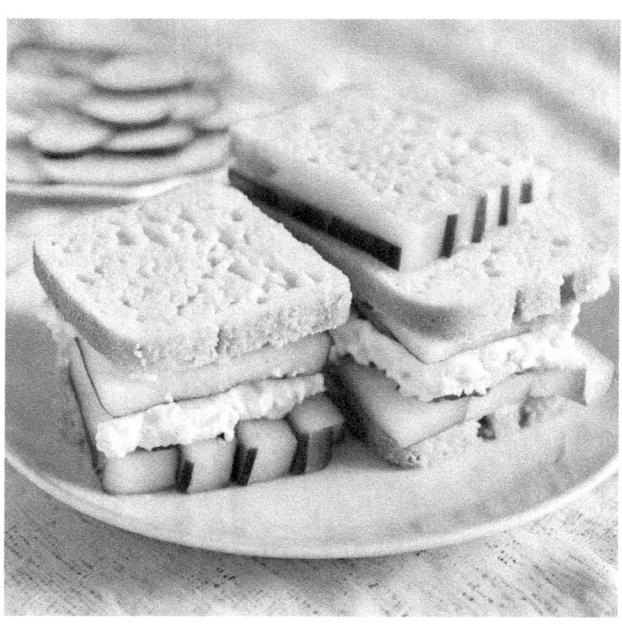

2. Summer Rice Salad

Ingredients:
- 1 cup cooked white rice
- 1/2 cup chopped bell peppers
- 1/2 cup chopped cucumber
- 1/4 cup chopped red onion
- 1/4 cup corn kernels
- 2 tablespoons olive oil
- 1 tablespoon apple cider vinegar
- 1 teaspoon dried basil

Instructions:
1. In a large bowl, combine the cooked rice with bell peppers, cucumber, red onion, and corn.
2. In a small bowl, whisk together olive oil, apple cider vinegar, and basil.
3. Pour the dressing over the rice mixture and stir well to combine.
4. Chill in the refrigerator for at least 30 minutes before serving to allow flavors to meld.

Nutrition Info Per Serving:
- Calories: 220
- Protein: 4 g
- Carbohydrates: 38 g
- Fat: 7 g
- Sodium: 10 mg
- Potassium: 150 mg
- Phosphorus: 80 mg

Serves: 4 **Preparation Time:** 40 minutes

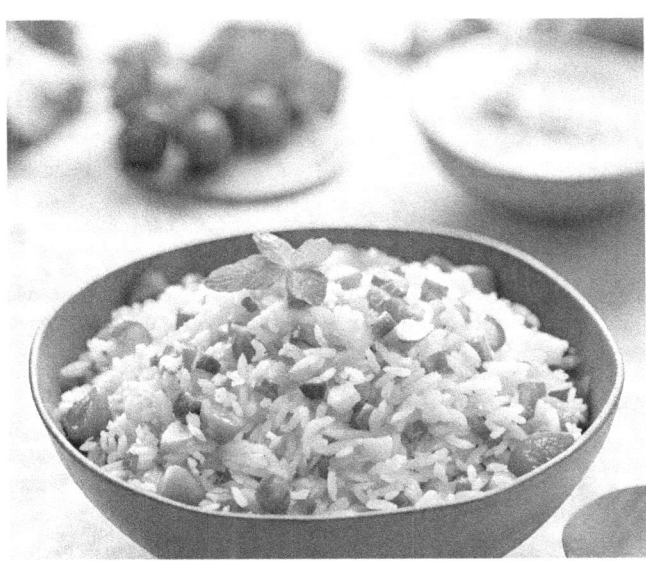

3. Pasta Salad

Ingredients:
- 2 cups cooked penne pasta
- 1 cup cherry tomatoes, halved
- 1/2 cup sliced black olives
- 1/4 cup diced green bell pepper
- 1/4 cup olive oil
- 2 tablespoons white wine vinegar
- 1 teaspoon dried oregano

Instructions:
1. In a large bowl, combine the cooked pasta, cherry tomatoes, black olives, and green bell pepper.
2. In a small bowl, whisk together olive oil, white wine vinegar, and oregano.
3. Pour the dressing over the pasta mixture and toss well to coat.
4. Refrigerate for at least 1 hour before serving to enhance the flavors.

Nutrition Info Per Serving:
- Calories: 290
- Protein: 7 g
- Carbohydrates: 45 g
- Fat: 10 g
- Sodium: 90 mg
- Potassium: 200 mg
- Phosphorus: 100 mg

Serves: 4 **Preparation Time:** 1 hour 15 minutes

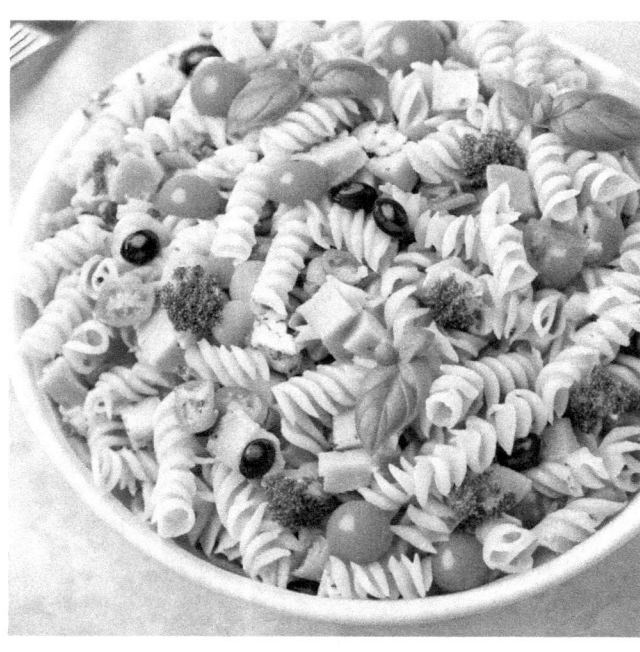

4. Vegetable Stir-Fry

Ingredients:
- 1 tablespoon olive oil
- 1 cup sliced carrots
- 1 cup sliced bell peppers
- 1 cup broccoli florets
- 1/2 cup sliced onions
- 2 cloves garlic, minced
- 2 tablespoons soy sauce (low sodium)
- 1 teaspoon sesame oil

Instructions:
1. Heat olive oil in a large skillet over medium heat.
2. Add carrots, bell peppers, broccoli, and onions. Stir-fry for about 5 minutes.
3. Add minced garlic and continue to stir-fry until vegetables are tender but still crisp, about 3-5 more minutes.
4. Drizzle with low sodium soy sauce and sesame oil, toss to combine, and serve hot.

Nutrition Info Per Serving:
- Calories: 120
- Protein: 3 g
- Carbohydrates: 15 g
- Fat: 6 g
- Sodium: 200 mg
- Potassium: 300 mg
- Phosphorus: 60 mg

Serves: 4 **Cooking Time:** 15 minutes

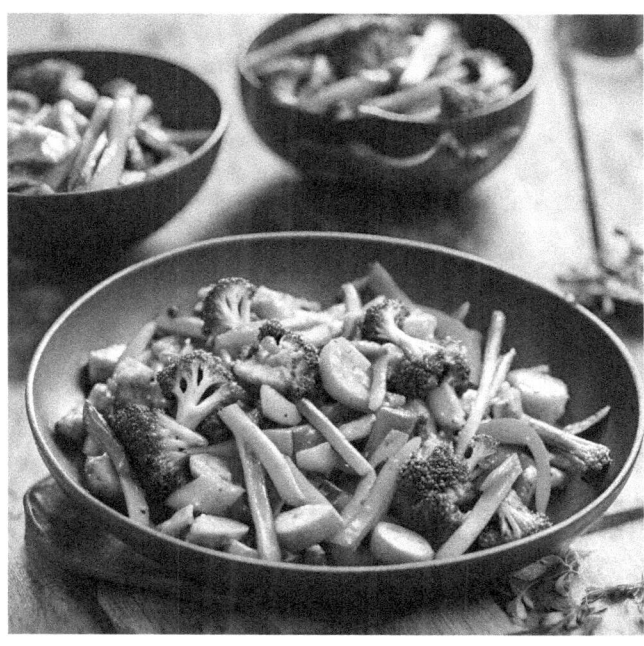

5. Beetroot and Onion Salad

Ingredients:
- 2 medium beetroots, cooked and sliced
- 1 small red onion, thinly sliced
- 2 tablespoons olive oil
- 1 tablespoon balsamic vinegar
- 1 teaspoon dried mint

Instructions:
1. In a salad bowl, combine sliced beetroots and red onion.
2. In a small bowl, whisk together olive oil, balsamic vinegar, and dried mint.
3. Drizzle the dressing over the beetroot and onion mixture and toss gently to coat.
4. Chill in the refrigerator for at least 30 minutes before serving to allow flavors to blend.

Nutrition Info Per Serving:
- Calories: 120
- Protein: 2 g
- Carbohydrates: 14 g
- Fat: 7 g
- Sodium: 55 mg
- Potassium: 267 mg
- Phosphorus: 37 mg

Serves: 4 **Preparation Time:** 40 minutes

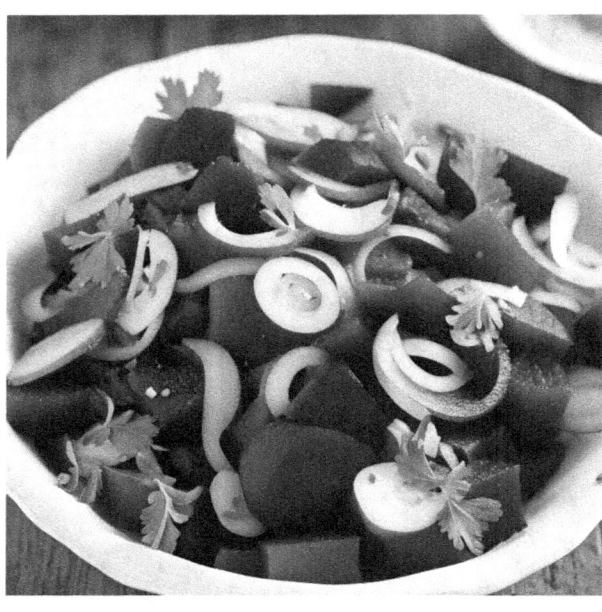

6. Mushroom Soup

Ingredients:
- 2 cups sliced mushrooms
- 1 tablespoon olive oil
- 1 small onion, chopped
- 2 cloves garlic, minced
- 3 cups vegetable broth (low sodium)
- 1/2 cup cream (or a non-dairy alternative)
- 1 teaspoon thyme

Instructions:
1. In a large pot, heat olive oil over medium heat. Add onions and garlic, and sauté until soft.
2. Add mushrooms and cook until they start to release their juices.
3. Pour in vegetable broth and bring to a simmer.
4. Add thyme and continue to simmer for about 20 minutes.
5. Blend the soup with an immersion blender until smooth.
6. Stir in cream and heat through.
7. Serve hot.

Nutrition Info Per Serving:
- Calories: 130
- Protein: 3 g
- Carbohydrates: 12 g
- Fat: 8 g
- Sodium: 75 mg
- Potassium: 300 mg
- Phosphorus: 50 mg

Serves: 4 **Cooking Time:** 30 minutes

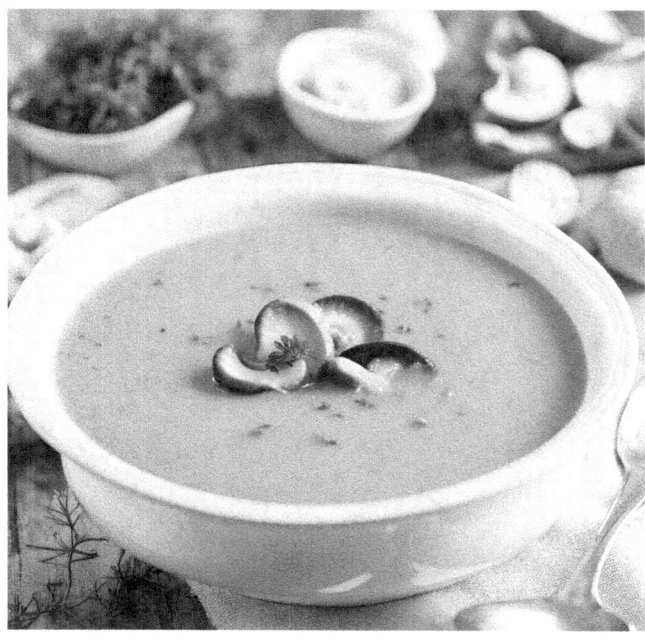

7. Rice Paper Rolls

Ingredients:
- 8 rice paper wrappers
- 1 cup cooked shrimp, peeled and halved
- 1 cup vermicelli noodles, cooked
- 1 cup lettuce, shredded
- 1 carrot, julienned
- 1/4 cup fresh mint leaves
- 1/4 cup fresh cilantro
- Dipping sauce (low sodium soy sauce mixed with a splash of lime juice and honey)

Instructions:
1. Dip one rice paper wrapper at a time in warm water until soft.
2. Place on a clean surface and in the center, layer some vermicelli noodles, lettuce, carrot, mint, cilantro, and shrimp.
3. Fold the bottom of the rice paper over the filling, then fold in sides and roll tightly.
4. Repeat with remaining wrappers and fillings.
5. Serve with dipping sauce.

Nutrition Info Per Serving:
- Calories: 150
- Protein: 10 g
- Carbohydrates: 20 g
- Fat: 2 g
- Sodium: 100 mg
- Potassium: 200 mg
- Phosphorus: 120 mg

Serves: 4 **Preparation Time:** 20 minutes

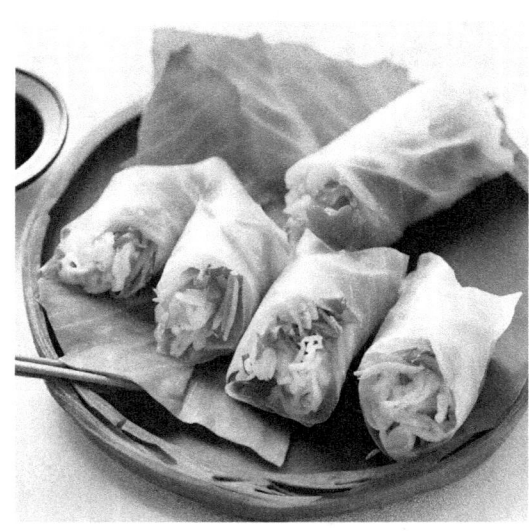

8. Egg Salad

Ingredients:
- 4 hard-boiled eggs, peeled and chopped
- 2 tablespoons mayonnaise (low fat)
- 1 tablespoon mustard
- 1/4 cup celery, finely chopped
- 1/4 cup red bell pepper, finely chopped
- Fresh herbs (such as dill or parsley), chopped

Instructions:
1. In a bowl, combine chopped eggs, mayonnaise, mustard, celery, red bell pepper, and fresh herbs.
2. Mix gently until all ingredients are well coated with mayonnaise.
3. Serve chilled on whole wheat bread or over a bed of lettuce.

Nutrition Info Per Serving:
- Calories: 140
- Protein: 7 g
- Carbohydrates: 3 g
- Fat: 11 g
- Sodium: 125 mg
- Potassium: 125 mg
- Phosphorus: 95 mg

Serves: 4 **Preparation Time:** 10 minutes

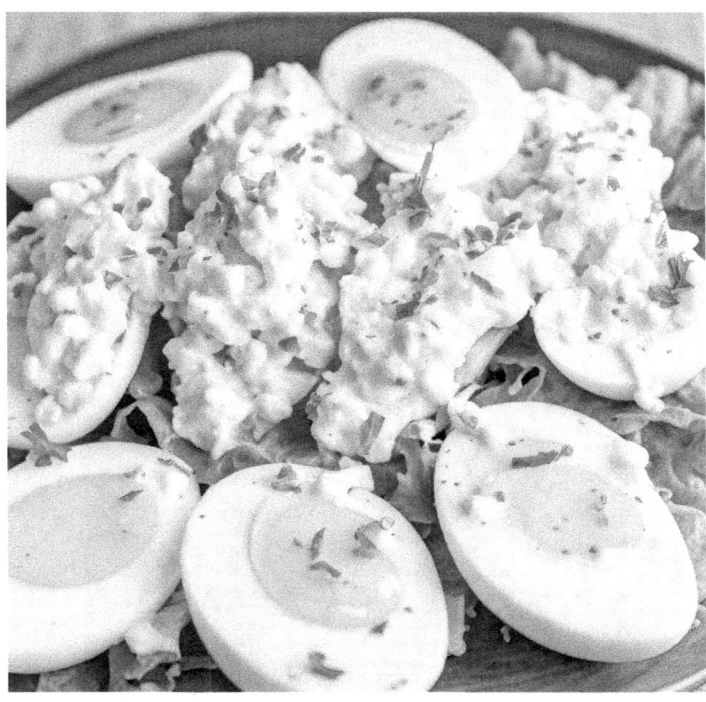

9. Roasted Bell Pepper Soup

Ingredients:
- 4 red bell peppers, halved and seeded
- 1 onion, chopped
- 2 cloves garlic, minced
- 3 cups vegetable broth (low sodium)
- 1 teaspoon smoked paprika
- 1/2 cup cream (or a non-dairy alternative)

Instructions:
1. Preheat the oven to 400°F (200°C). Place bell peppers cut-side down on a baking sheet and roast until skins are blistered and blackened, about 25-30 minutes.
2. Remove from oven, cover with a kitchen towel, and let cool. Peel off the skins.
3. In a pot, heat a splash of olive oil over medium heat. Add onion and garlic, and sauté until soft.
4. Add roasted bell peppers, vegetable broth, and smoked paprika. Bring to a simmer and cook for 15 minutes.
5. Blend the soup until smooth. Stir in cream and heat through.
6. Serve hot.

Nutrition Info Per Serving:
- Calories: 150
- Protein: 2 g
- Carbohydrates: 15 g
- Fat: 9 g
- Sodium: 75 mg
- Potassium: 250 mg
- Phosphorus: 50 mg

Serves: 4 **Cooking Time:** 55 minutes

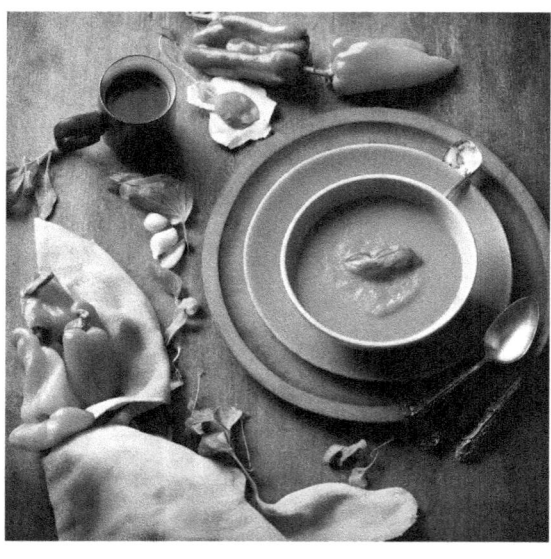

10. Pita Pockets

Ingredients:
- 2 whole wheat pita breads, halved
- 1 cup cooked chicken breast, chopped
- 1/2 cup cucumber, diced
- 1/2 cup tomatoes, diced
- 1/4 cup low-fat Greek yogurt
- 1 tablespoon fresh mint, chopped
- 1 teaspoon lemon juice

Instructions:
1. In a bowl, mix together the Greek yogurt, mint, and lemon juice.
2. Stir in the chicken, cucumber, and tomatoes until well combined.
3. Spoon the mixture into each pita half.
4. Serve immediately or chill until ready to serve.

Nutrition Info Per Serving:
- Calories: 220
- Protein: 18 g
- Carbohydrates: 26 g
- Fat: 5 g
- Sodium: 160 mg
- Potassium: 300 mg
- Phosphorus: 150 mg

Serves: 4 **Preparation Time:** 15 minutes

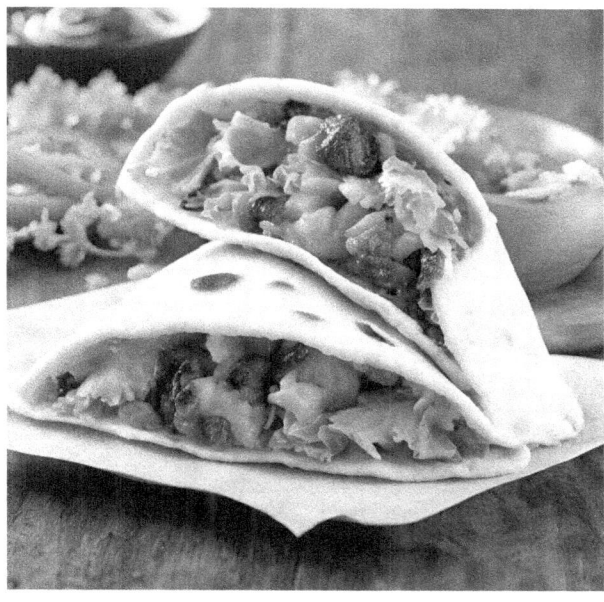

11. Celery Sticks with Hummus

Ingredients:
- 1 cup hummus (homemade or store-bought with low sodium)
- 8 celery sticks, washed and cut into 3-4 inch pieces

Instructions:
1. Spoon hummus into a serving bowl.
2. Arrange celery sticks around the bowl for dipping.
3. Serve immediately or cover and chill until ready to serve.

Nutrition Info Per Serving:
- Calories: 100
- Protein: 5 g
- Carbohydrates: 8 g
- Fat: 6 g
- Sodium: 120 mg
- Potassium: 115 mg
- Phosphorus: 60 mg

Serves: 4 **Preparation Time:** 10 minutes

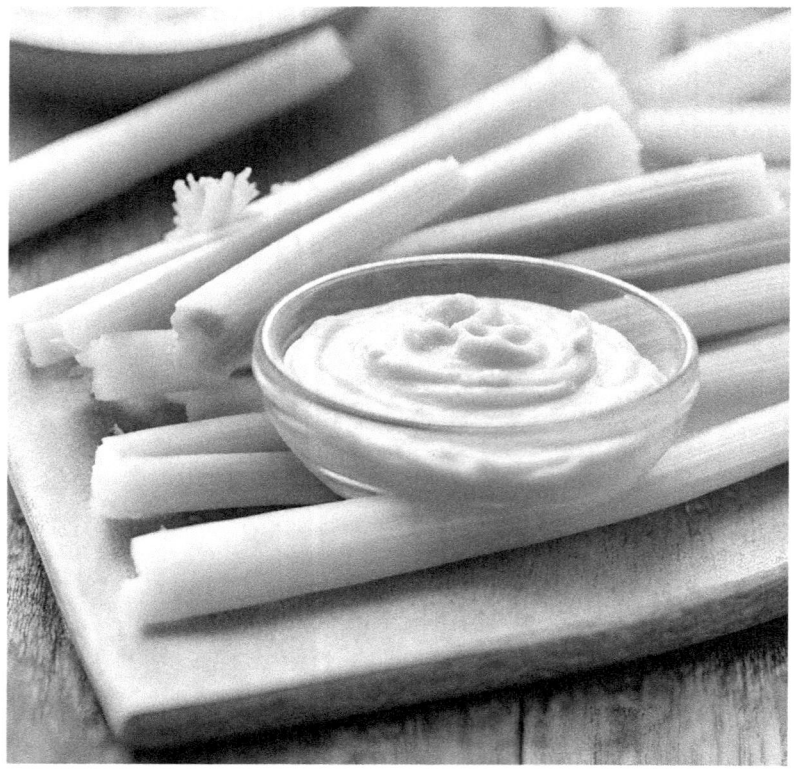

12. Carrot Ginger Soup

Ingredients:
- 4 large carrots, peeled and chopped
- 1 tablespoon fresh ginger, minced
- 1 onion, chopped
- 4 cups vegetable broth (low sodium)
- 1 tablespoon olive oil
- 1/2 cup coconut milk

Instructions:
1. In a large pot, heat olive oil over medium heat.
2. Add onion and ginger, sauté until the onion becomes translucent.
3. Add the chopped carrots and cook for about 5 minutes, stirring occasionally.
4. Pour in the vegetable broth and bring to a boil.
5. Reduce heat to low, cover, and simmer until carrots are tender, about 20 minutes.
6. Use an immersion blender to puree the soup until smooth.
7. Stir in coconut milk and heat through.
8. Serve hot.

Nutrition Info Per Serving:
- Calories: 150
- Protein: 2 g
- Carbohydrates: 18 g
- Fat: 8 g
- Sodium: 100 mg
- Potassium: 350 mg
- Phosphorus: 50 mg

Serves: 4 **Cooking Time:** 35 minutes

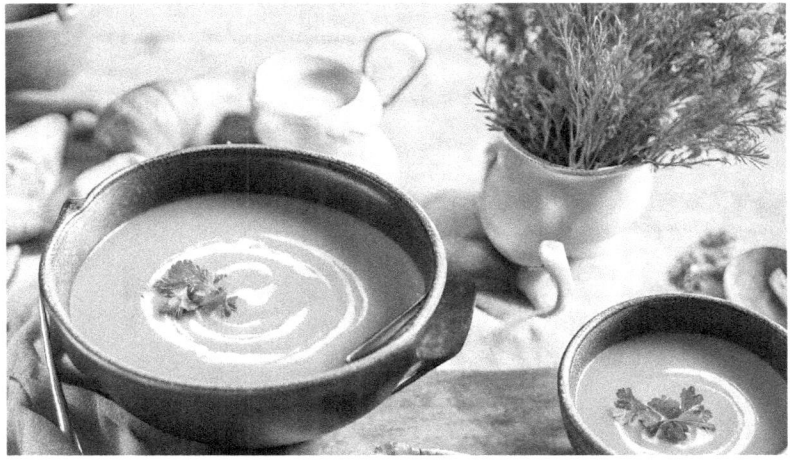

13. Cauliflower Steak

Ingredients:
- 1 large head cauliflower
- 2 tablespoons olive oil
- 1 teaspoon garlic powder
- 1 teaspoon paprika
- Fresh herbs for garnish (such as parsley or thyme)

Instructions:
1. Preheat oven to 400°F (200°C).
2. Slice cauliflower into 1-inch thick steaks.
3. Place cauliflower steaks on a baking sheet.
4. Brush both sides of each steak with olive oil and sprinkle with garlic powder and paprika.
5. Roast in the oven for about 25 minutes or until golden brown and tender.
6. Garnish with fresh herbs before serving.

Nutrition Info Per Serving:
- Calories: 120
- Protein: 4 g
- Carbohydrates: 10 g
- Fat: 8 g
- Sodium: 45 mg
- Potassium: 450 mg
- Phosphorus: 44 mg

Serves: 4 **Cooking Time:** 30 minutes

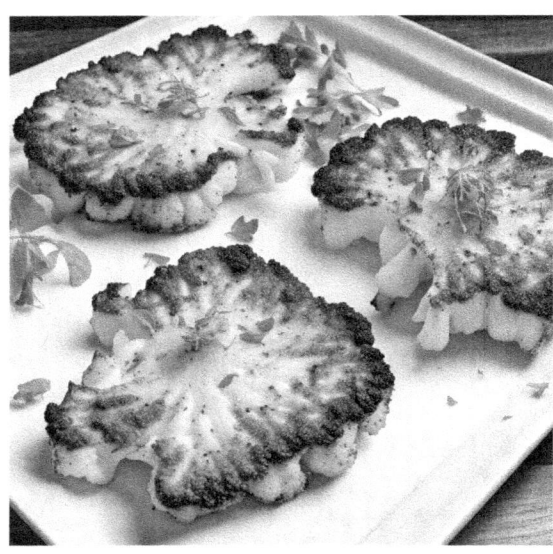

14. Parsley and Lemon Pasta

Ingredients:
- 200 grams spaghetti (whole wheat, if available)
- 1/4 cup olive oil
- 3 cloves garlic, minced
- Zest and juice of 1 lemon
- 1/4 cup chopped fresh parsley
- 1/4 cup grated Parmesan cheese (optional)

Instructions:
1. Cook pasta according to package instructions until al dente; drain.
2. In the same pot, heat olive oil over medium heat.
3. Add garlic and cook until fragrant, about 1 minute.
4. Add the cooked pasta back to the pot along with lemon zest, lemon juice, and parsley.
5. Toss until the pasta is well coated.
6. Serve topped with grated Parmesan if desired.

Nutrition Info Per Serving:
- Calories: 310
- Protein: 8 g
- Carbohydrates: 42 g
- Fat: 12 g
- Sodium: 85 mg
- Potassium: 125 mg
- Phosphorus: 90 mg

Serves: 4 **Cooking Time:** 20 minutes

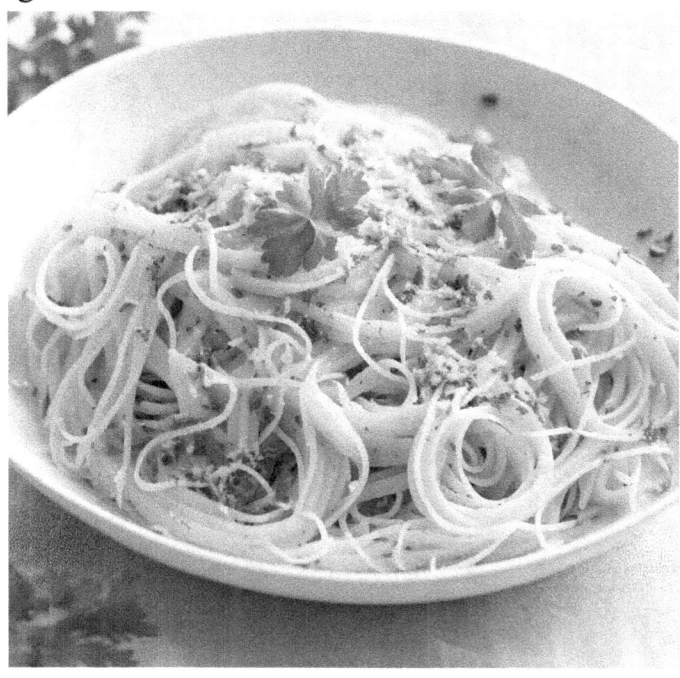

15. Mixed Berry Salad

Ingredients:
- 1 cup strawberries, hulled and halved
- 1 cup blueberries
- 1 cup raspberries
- 1 cup blackberries
- 2 tablespoons honey
- 1 teaspoon lemon zest
- 1 tablespoon lemon juice
- Fresh mint leaves for garnish

Instructions:
1. In a large bowl, combine all the berries.
2. In a small bowl, whisk together honey, lemon zest, and lemon juice.
3. Drizzle the dressing over the berries and gently toss to coat.
4. Garnish with fresh mint leaves before serving.

Nutrition Info Per Serving:
- Calories: 120
- Protein: 2 g
- Carbohydrates: 28 g
- Fat: 0.5 g
- Sodium: 5 mg
- Potassium: 180 mg
- Phosphorus: 35 mg

Serves: 4 **Preparation Time:** 10 minutes

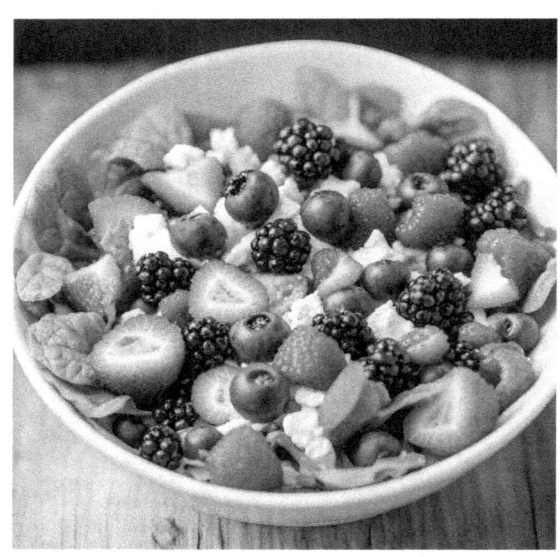

16. Garlic Mashed Potatoes

Ingredients:
- 4 medium potatoes, peeled and cubed
- 3 cloves garlic, minced
- 1/4 cup milk (or non-dairy alternative)
- 2 tablespoons olive oil
- Fresh chives, chopped for garnish

Instructions:
1. Place the potatoes in a pot and cover with water. Bring to a boil, then reduce heat and simmer until tender, about 20 minutes.
2. Drain the potatoes and return them to the pot.
3. Add minced garlic, milk, and olive oil.
4. Mash the potatoes until smooth and creamy.
5. Garnish with chopped chives before serving.

Nutrition Info Per Serving:
- Calories: 220
- Protein: 4 g
- Carbohydrates: 35 g
- Fat: 7 g
- Sodium: 30 mg
- Potassium: 750 mg
- Phosphorus: 70 mg

Serves: 4 **Cooking Time:** 30 minutes

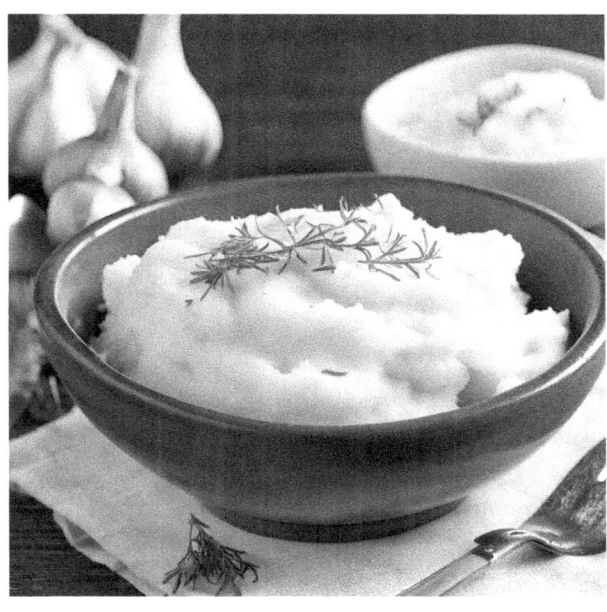

17. Vegetable Kabobs

Ingredients:
- 1 zucchini, cut into chunks
- 1 yellow squash, cut into chunks
- 1 red bell pepper, cut into chunks
- 1 onion, cut into chunks
- 2 tablespoons olive oil
- 1 teaspoon dried oregano

Instructions:
1. Preheat the grill to medium-high heat.
2. Thread the vegetables onto skewers.
3. Brush with olive oil and sprinkle with oregano.
4. Grill, turning occasionally, until vegetables are tender and slightly charred, about 10-15 minutes.
5. Serve hot.

Nutrition Info Per Serving:
- Calories: 110
- Protein: 2 g
- Carbohydrates: 10 g
- Fat: 7 g
- Sodium: 10 mg
- Potassium: 300 mg
- Phosphorus: 50 mg

Serves: 4 **Cooking Time:** 15 minutes

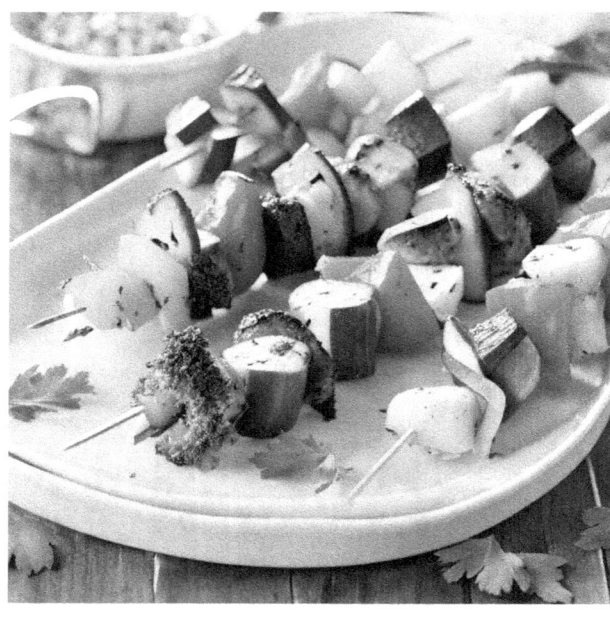

18. Cornflake Cereal with Almond Milk

Ingredients:
- 1 cup cornflakes
- 1 cup almond milk

Instructions:
1. Pour cornflakes into a bowl.
2. Add almond milk.
3. Serve immediately to maintain crunchiness.

Nutrition Info Per Serving:
- Calories: 150
- Protein: 2 g
- Carbohydrates: 29 g
- Fat: 3 g
- Sodium: 200 mg
- Potassium: 90 mg
- Phosphorus: 50 mg

Serves: 1 **Preparation Time:** 2 minutes

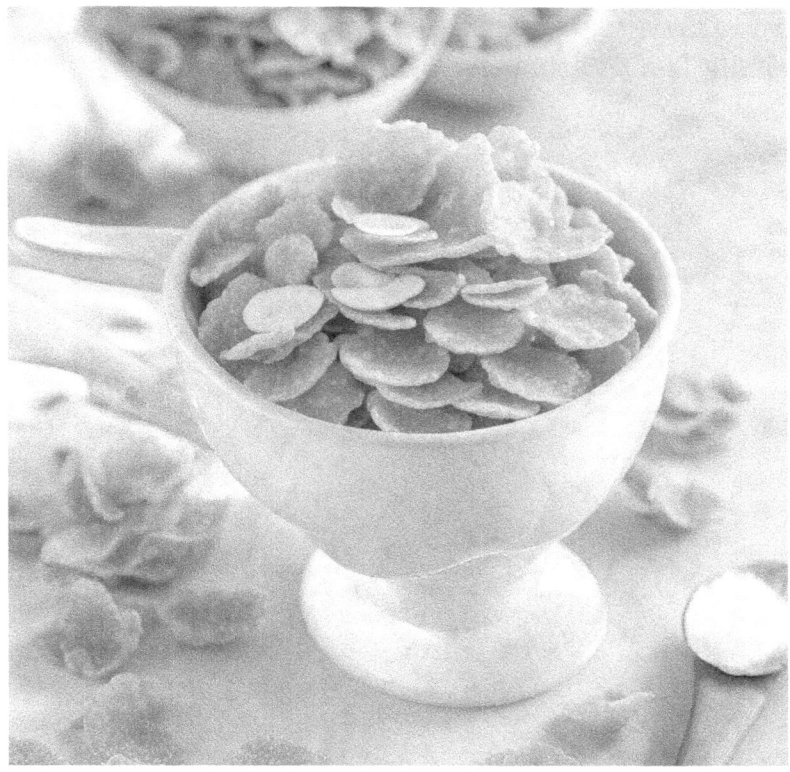

19. Poached Eggs on Baby Kale

Ingredients:
- 2 eggs
- 2 cups baby kale
- 1 teaspoon olive oil
- 1 tablespoon vinegar (for poaching)

Instructions:
1. Bring a pot of water to a gentle simmer and add vinegar.
2. Crack eggs into the water and poach for 3-4 minutes until whites are set but yolks remain runny.
3. Meanwhile, sauté baby kale in olive oil until wilted.
4. Serve poached eggs on top of sautéed kale.

Nutrition Info Per Serving:
- Calories: 140
- Protein: 10 g
- Carbohydrates: 3 g
- Fat: 10 g
- Sodium: 125 mg
- Potassium: 400 mg
- Phosphorus: 185 mg

Serves: 2 **Cooking Time:** 10 minutes

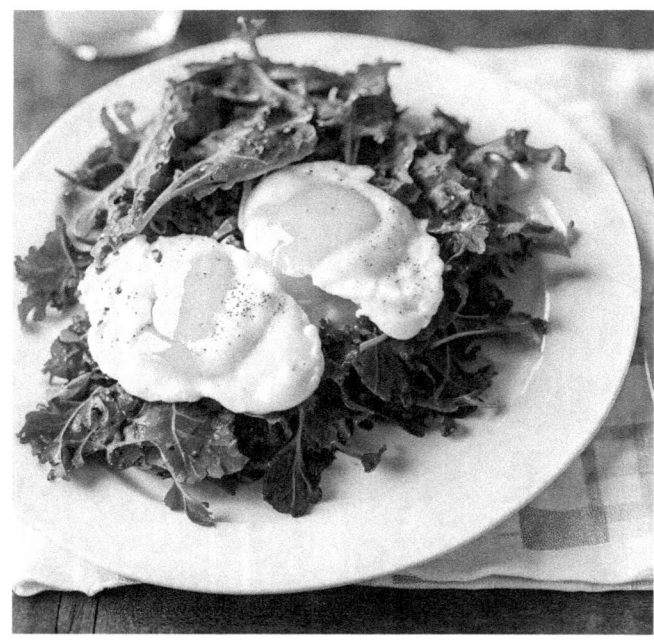

20. Apple Cinnamon Pancakes

Ingredients:
- 1 cup whole wheat flour
- 1 tablespoon sugar
- 2 teaspoons baking powder
- 1/2 teaspoon cinnamon
- 1 cup milk (or non-dairy alternative)
- 1 egg
- 1 apple, peeled and grated
- 1 teaspoon vanilla extract

Instructions:
1. In a large bowl, mix together flour, sugar, baking powder, and cinnamon.
2. In another bowl, whisk together milk, egg, and vanilla extract.
3. Stir the wet ingredients into the dry ingredients until just combined.
4. Fold in the grated apple.
5. Heat a non-stick skillet over medium heat and lightly grease it.
6. Pour 1/4 cup of batter for each pancake and cook until bubbles form on the surface, then flip and cook until golden brown on the other side.
7. Serve warm.

Nutrition Info Per Serving:
- Calories: 210
- Protein: 6 g
- Carbohydrates: 38 g
- Fat: 4 g
- Sodium: 240 mg
- Potassium: 200 mg
- Phosphorus: 180 mg

Serves: 4 **Cooking Time:** 20 minutes

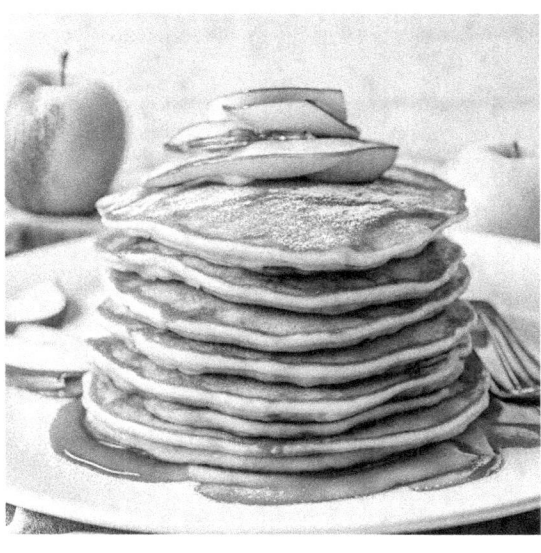

21. Asparagus Spears

Ingredients:
- 1 pound asparagus, trimmed
- 2 teaspoons olive oil
- 1 lemon, zested and juiced

Instructions:
1. Preheat the oven to 400°F (200°C).
2. Arrange asparagus on a baking sheet.
3. Drizzle with olive oil and lemon juice.
4. Roast in the oven until tender, about 15-20 minutes.
5. Sprinkle with lemon zest before serving.

Nutrition Info Per Serving:
- Calories: 60
- Protein: 3 g
- Carbohydrates: 5 g
- Fat: 3.5 g
- Sodium: 2 mg
- Potassium: 230 mg
- Phosphorus: 50 mg

Serves: 4 **Cooking Time:** 20 minutes

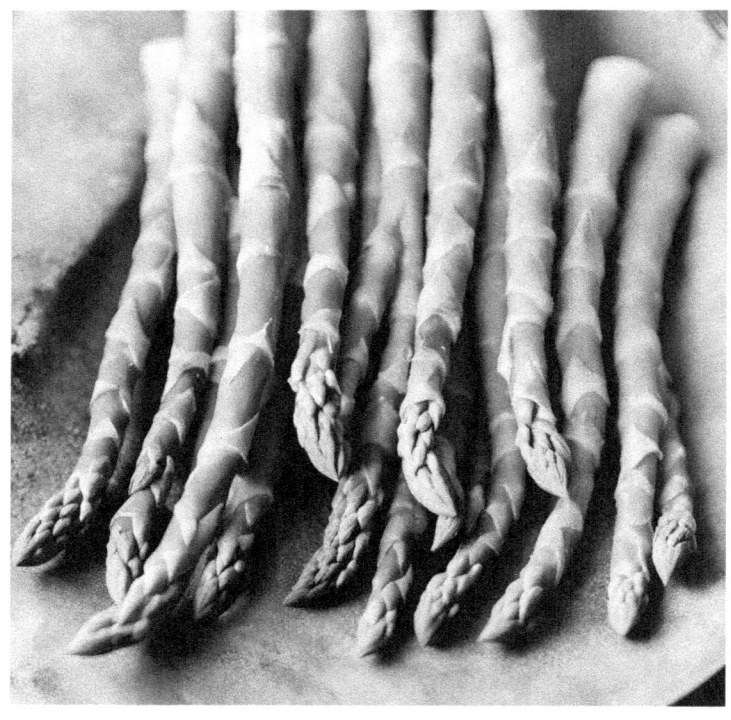

22. Spaghetti Squash with Tomato Sauce

Ingredients:
- 1 spaghetti squash, halved lengthwise and seeds removed
- 2 cups crushed tomatoes
- 1 onion, chopped
- 2 cloves garlic, minced
- 1 teaspoon dried basil
- 1 teaspoon dried oregano
- 1 tablespoon olive oil

Instructions:
1. Preheat the oven to 375°F (190°C).
2. Place spaghetti squash halves cut-side down on a baking sheet and bake until tender, about 40-45 minutes.
3. While the squash is baking, heat olive oil in a saucepan over medium heat.
4. Add onion and garlic, and sauté until soft.
5. Add crushed tomatoes, basil, and oregano. Simmer for 20 minutes.
6. Once squash is done, use a fork to scrape the inside, creating spaghetti-like strands.
7. Serve the tomato sauce over the spaghetti squash strands.

Nutrition Info Per Serving:
- Calories: 150
- Protein: 3 g
- Carbohydrates: 20 g
- Fat: 7 g
- Sodium: 10 mg
- Potassium: 400 mg
- Phosphorus: 70 mg

Serves: 4 **Cooking Time:** 1 hour 5 minutes

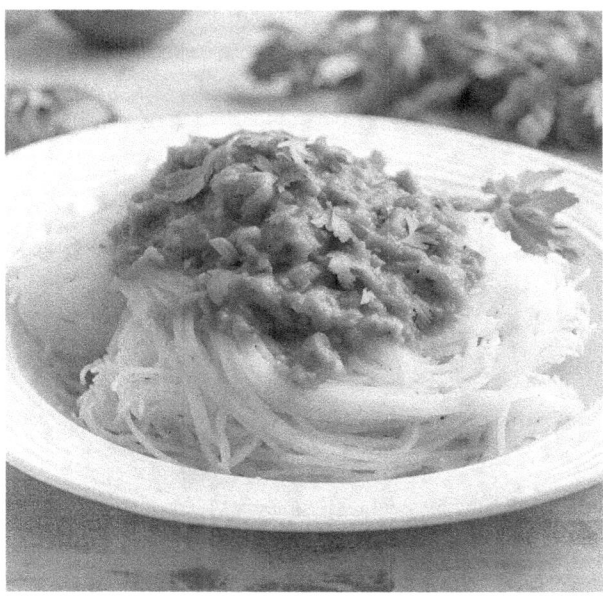

Dinner Recipes

1. Grilled Zucchini and Squash
Ingredients:
- 2 zucchinis, sliced lengthwise
- 2 yellow squashes, sliced lengthwise
- 2 tablespoons olive oil
- 1 teaspoon dried thyme

Instructions:
1. Preheat grill to medium-high heat.
2. Brush both sides of the zucchini and squash slices with olive oil and sprinkle with thyme.
3. Grill for 4-5 minutes on each side or until tender and grill marks appear.
4. Serve hot.

Nutrition Info Per Serving:
- Calories: 120
- Protein: 2 g
- Carbohydrates: 8 g
- Fat: 9 g
- Sodium: 10 mg
- Potassium: 510 mg
- Phosphorus: 70 mg

Serves: 4 **Cooking Time:** 10 minutes

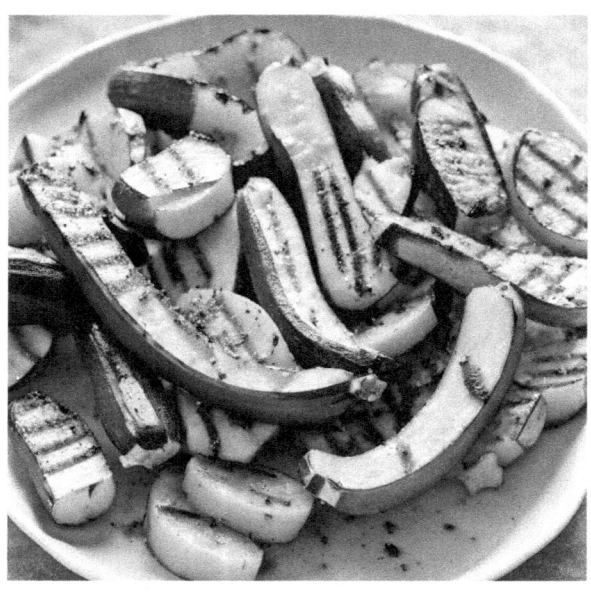

2. Cabbage Stir-Fry

Ingredients:
- 1 head of cabbage, shredded
- 1 carrot, julienned
- 1 bell pepper, sliced
- 2 tablespoons olive oil
- 1 tablespoon vinegar
- 1 teaspoon garlic, minced

Instructions:
1. Heat olive oil in a large skillet over medium-high heat.
2. Add garlic and sauté for about 1 minute until fragrant.
3. Add the shredded cabbage, carrot, and bell pepper to the skillet.
4. Stir-fry for 5-7 minutes until vegetables are tender.
5. Drizzle with vinegar and toss to combine.
6. Serve hot.

Nutrition Info Per Serving:
- Calories: 110
- Protein: 2 g
- Carbohydrates: 13 g
- Fat: 6 g
- Sodium: 30 mg
- Potassium: 320 mg
- Phosphorus: 49 mg

Serves: 4 **Cooking Time:** 10 minutes

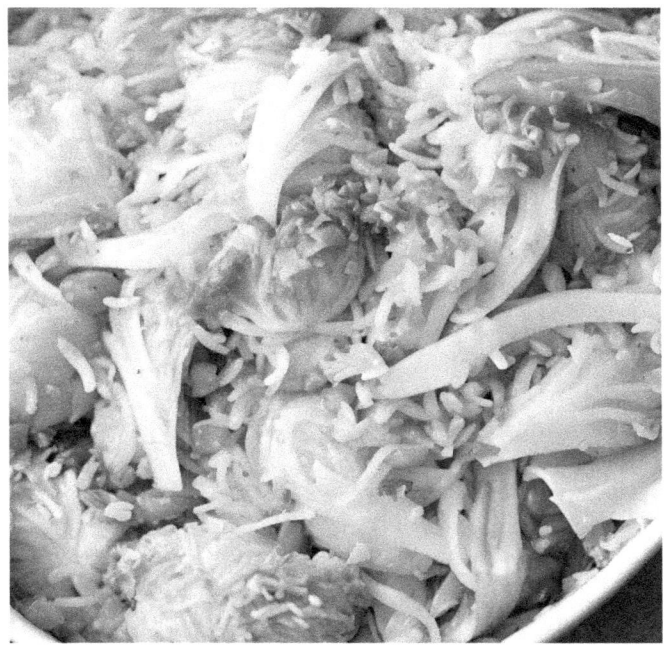

3. Carrot Risotto

Ingredients:
- 1 cup Arborio rice
- 4 cups low-sodium vegetable broth
- 1 onion, finely chopped
- 2 carrots, grated
- 2 tablespoons olive oil
- 1/4 cup Parmesan cheese, grated (optional)
- 1 tablespoon fresh parsley, chopped

Instructions:
1. Heat olive oil in a large saucepan over medium heat.
2. Add onion and sauté until translucent.
3. Stir in Arborio rice and cook for 2 minutes, stirring constantly.
4. Gradually add vegetable broth, one cup at a time, stirring frequently until each cup is absorbed before adding the next.
5. When the rice is almost cooked, stir in grated carrots.
6. Continue cooking until the rice is creamy and tender.
7. Remove from heat and stir in Parmesan cheese if using and parsley.
8. Serve immediately.

Nutrition Info Per Serving:
- Calories: 250
- Protein: 5 g
- Carbohydrates: 45 g
- Fat: 7 g
- Sodium: 70 mg
- Potassium: 270 mg
- Phosphorus: 90 mg

Serves: 4 **Cooking Time:** 30 minutes

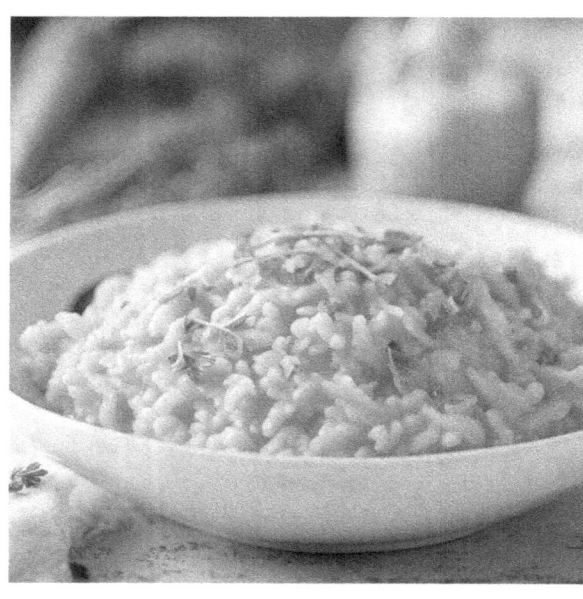

4. Garlic Butter Baked Tilapia

Ingredients:
- 4 tilapia fillets
- 4 tablespoons unsalted butter, melted
- 2 cloves garlic, minced
- 1 tablespoon lemon juice
- Fresh parsley, chopped for garnish

Instructions:
1. Preheat oven to 400°F (200°C).
2. Place tilapia fillets in a baking dish.
3. In a small bowl, combine melted butter, garlic, and lemon juice.
4. Pour the butter mixture over the tilapia.
5. Bake in the preheated oven for 12-15 minutes, or until fish flakes easily with a fork.
6. Garnish with chopped parsley before serving.

Nutrition Info Per Serving:
- Calories: 220
- Protein: 23 g
- Carbohydrates: 1 g
- Fat: 14 g
- Sodium: 90 mg
- Potassium: 330 mg
- Phosphorus: 170 mg

Serves: 4 **Cooking Time:** 15 minutes

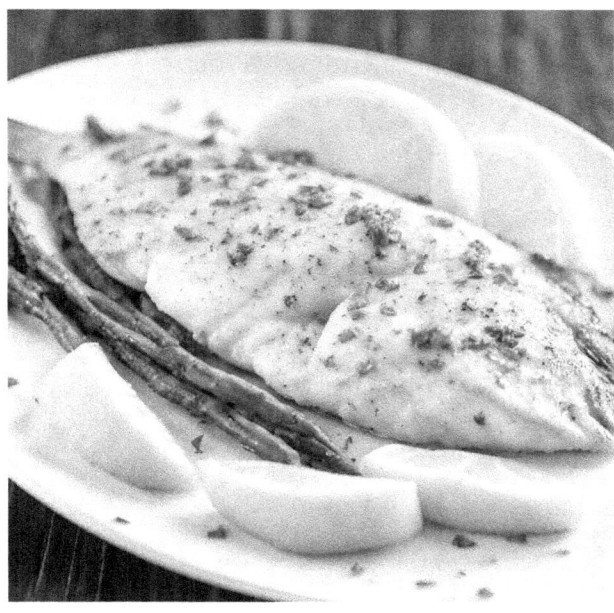

5. Baked Apple and Fennel

Ingredients:
- 2 large apples, cored and sliced
- 1 fennel bulb, sliced
- 2 tablespoons olive oil
- 1 teaspoon dried thyme
- 1/4 cup apple juice

Instructions:
1. Preheat oven to 375°F (190°C).
2. In a baking dish, arrange the apple and fennel slices.
3. Drizzle with olive oil and sprinkle thyme over the top.
4. Pour apple juice into the bottom of the dish.
5. Bake in preheated oven for 25-30 minutes, or until fennel is tender and apples are lightly caramelized.
6. Serve warm.

Nutrition Info Per Serving:
- Calories: 160
- Protein: 1 g
- Carbohydrates: 23 g
- Fat: 8 g
- Sodium: 30 mg
- Potassium: 360 mg
- Phosphorus: 40 mg

Serves: 4 **Cooking Time:** 30 minutes

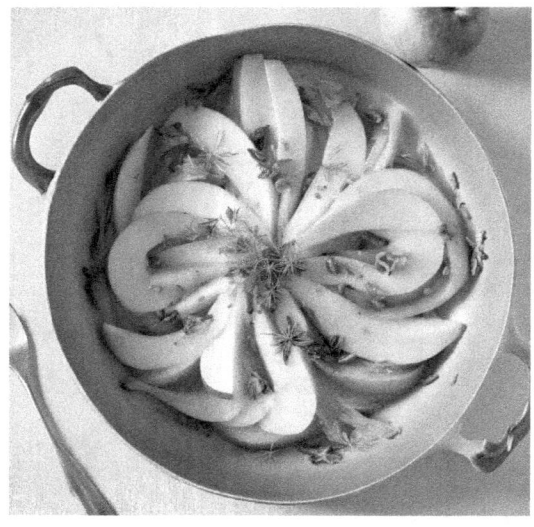

6. Herb-Roasted Potatoes

Ingredients:
- 4 medium potatoes, cubed
- 2 tablespoons olive oil
- 1 teaspoon dried rosemary
- 1 teaspoon dried thyme

Instructions:
1. Preheat oven to 400°F (200°C).
2. Toss potatoes with olive oil, rosemary, and thyme in a large bowl.
3. Spread the potatoes in a single layer on a baking sheet.
4. Roast for 30-35 minutes, stirring halfway through, until potatoes are golden and crisp.
5. Serve hot.

Nutrition Info Per Serving:
- Calories: 200
- Protein: 4 g
- Carbohydrates: 30 g
- Fat: 7 g
- Sodium: 20 mg
- Potassium: 715 mg
- Phosphorus: 75 mg

Serves: 4 **Cooking Time:** 35 minutes

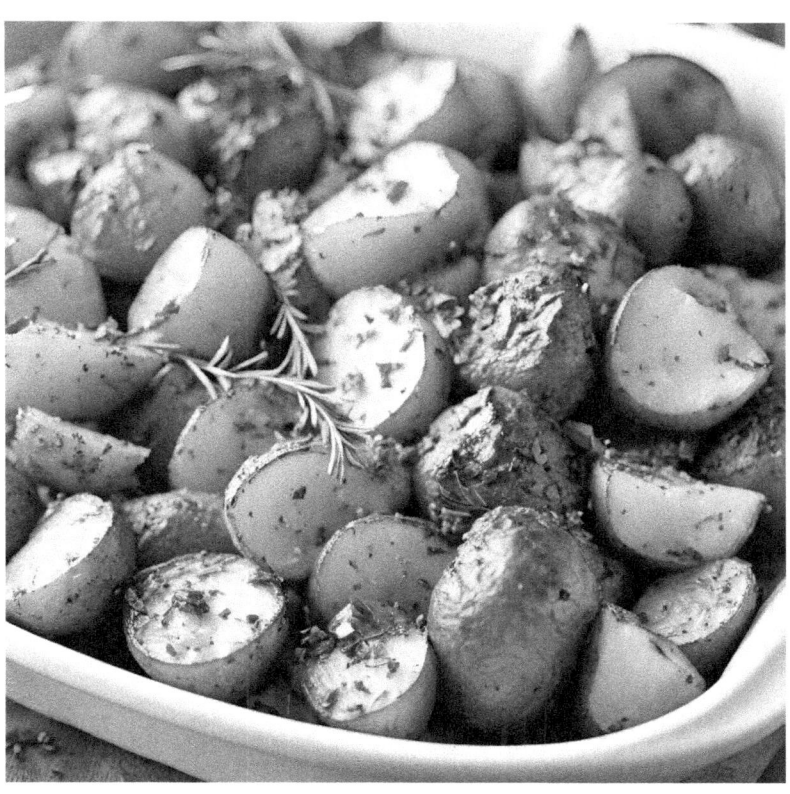

7. Mixed Vegetable Grill

Ingredients:
- 1 zucchini, sliced
- 1 yellow squash, sliced
- 1 red bell pepper, seeded and sliced
- 1 eggplant, sliced
- 2 tablespoons olive oil
- 1 teaspoon dried oregano

Instructions:
1. Preheat grill to medium-high heat.
2. Brush vegetables with olive oil and sprinkle with oregano.
3. Grill vegetables for about 3-4 minutes on each side or until tender and slightly charred.
4. Serve hot.

Nutrition Info Per Serving:
- Calories: 130
- Protein: 3 g
- Carbohydrates: 15 g
- Fat: 7 g
- Sodium: 10 mg
- Potassium: 450 mg
- Phosphorus: 50 mg

Serves: 4 **Cooking Time:** 10 minutes

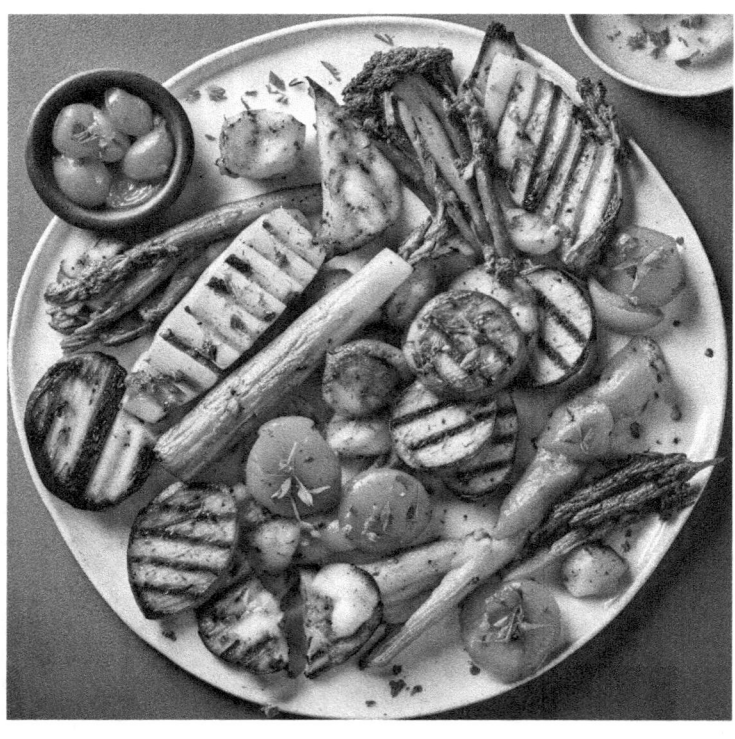

8. Cauliflower Soup

Ingredients:
- 1 head cauliflower, chopped
- 1 onion, chopped
- 2 cloves garlic, minced
- 4 cups low-sodium vegetable broth
- 1/4 cup cream (or non-dairy alternative)
- 2 tablespoons olive oil

Instructions:
1. In a large pot, heat olive oil over medium heat.
2. Add onion and garlic and sauté until onion is translucent.
3. Add cauliflower and vegetable broth; bring to a boil.
4. Reduce heat and simmer for 20 minutes or until cauliflower is tender.
5. Puree the soup with an immersion blender until smooth.
6. Stir in cream, heat through, and serve.

Nutrition Info Per Serving:
- Calories: 180
- Protein: 5 g
- Carbohydrates: 15 g
- Fat: 12 g
- Sodium: 55 mg
- Potassium: 470 mg
- Phosphorus: 80 mg

Serves: 4 **Cooking Time:** 30 minutes

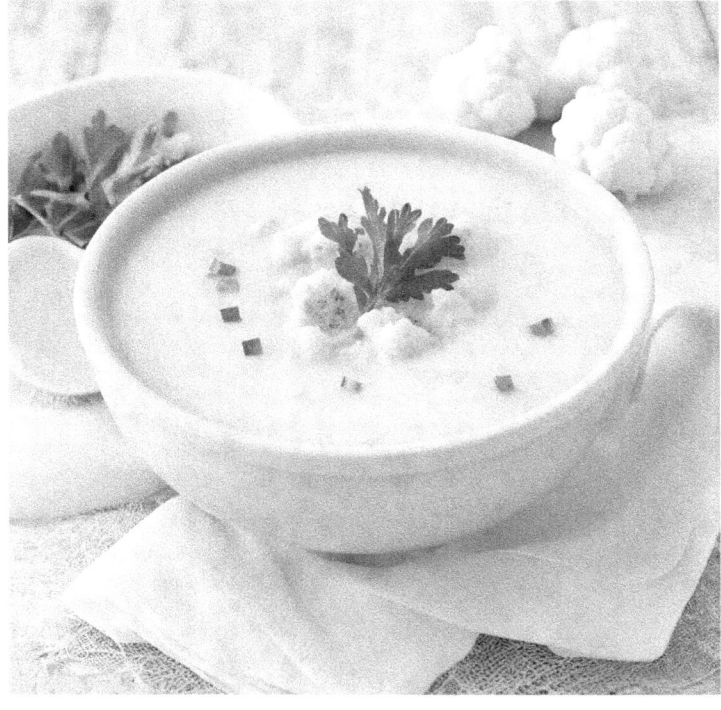

9. Egg White Frittata

Ingredients:
- 8 egg whites
- 1 cup spinach, chopped
- 1/2 cup mushrooms, sliced
- 1/2 cup red bell pepper, diced
- 1 onion, diced
- 2 tablespoons olive oil
- 1/4 cup low-fat milk
- Fresh herbs (like parsley or chives), chopped

Instructions:
1. Preheat oven to 375°F (190°C).
2. In a skillet, heat olive oil over medium heat.
3. Sauté onion, bell pepper, and mushrooms until softened.
4. Add spinach and cook until wilted.
5. In a large bowl, whisk together egg whites and milk. Stir in sautéed vegetables and fresh herbs.
6. Pour mixture into a greased baking dish.
7. Bake in the oven for 20-25 minutes, or until eggs are set and the top is slightly golden.
8. Serve hot.

Nutrition Info Per Serving:
- Calories: 130
- Protein: 11 g
- Carbohydrates: 8 g
- Fat: 6 g
- Sodium: 170 mg
- Potassium: 320 mg
- Phosphorus: 100 mg

Serves: 4 **Cooking Time:** 45 minutes

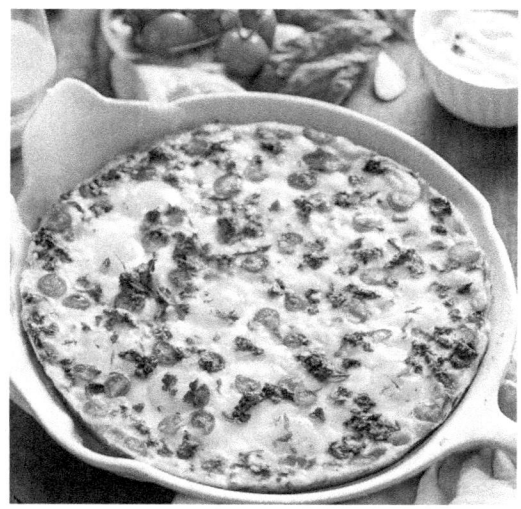

10. Stuffed Tomato with Rice

Ingredients:
- 4 large tomatoes
- 1 cup cooked rice
- 1/2 cup peas
- 1/2 cup corn
- 1/4 cup chopped onion
- 1 clove garlic, minced
- 2 tablespoons olive oil
- Fresh basil, chopped

Instructions:
1. Preheat oven to 350°F (175°C).
2. Cut the tops off the tomatoes and scoop out the insides, leaving a shell.
3. In a skillet, heat olive oil over medium heat. Sauté onion and garlic until translucent.
4. Stir in cooked rice, peas, and corn. Cook until heated through.
5. Spoon the rice mixture into the tomato shells.
6. Place stuffed tomatoes in a baking dish and bake for 20-25 minutes, until tomatoes are tender.
7. Garnish with fresh basil before serving.

Nutrition Info Per Serving:
- Calories: 200
- Protein: 4 g
- Carbohydrates: 30 g
- Fat: 7 g
- Sodium: 30 mg
- Potassium: 400 mg
- Phosphorus: 70 mg

Serves: 4 **Cooking Time:** 45 minutes

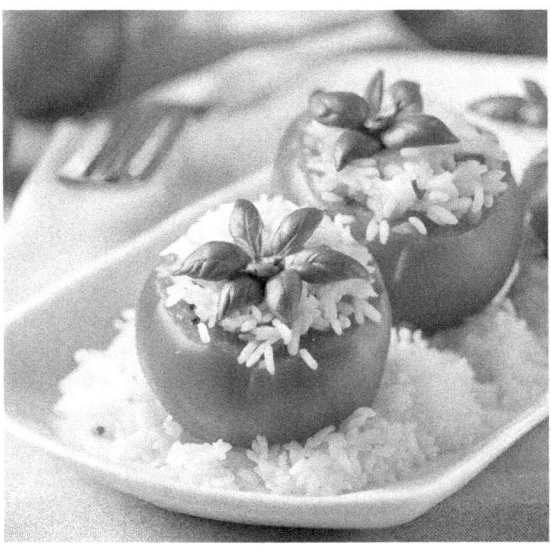

11. Pasta Primavera

Ingredients:
- 2 cups cooked whole wheat spaghetti
- 1/2 cup sliced zucchini
- 1/2 cup sliced carrots
- 1/2 cup broccoli florets
- 1/2 cup sliced bell peppers
- 1/4 cup olive oil
- 1/2 cup low-sodium vegetable broth
- 1 teaspoon dried Italian herbs
- Fresh parsley, chopped

Instructions:
1. In a large skillet, heat olive oil over medium heat.
2. Add zucchini, carrots, broccoli, and bell peppers. Sauté until vegetables are tender.
3. Add cooked spaghetti, vegetable broth, and Italian herbs. Toss well and heat through.
4. Garnish with chopped parsley before serving.

Nutrition Info Per Serving:
- Calories: 250
- Protein: 8 g
- Carbohydrates: 35 g
- Fat: 10 g
- Sodium: 55 mg
- Potassium: 350 mg
- Phosphorus: 90 mg

Serves: 4 **Cooking Time:** 30 minutes

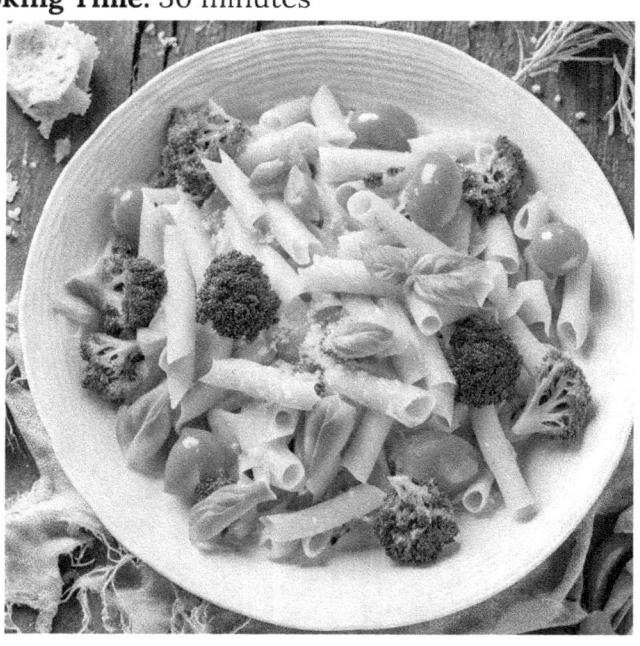

12. Garlic Spinach Sauté

Ingredients:
- 4 cups spinach leaves
- 3 cloves garlic, minced
- 2 tablespoons olive oil

Instructions:
1. Heat olive oil in a large skillet over medium heat.
2. Add minced garlic and sauté for about 1 minute until fragrant.
3. Add spinach leaves and cook until wilted, about 3-4 minutes.
4. Serve hot.

Nutrition Info Per Serving:
- Calories: 90
- Protein: 3 g
- Carbohydrates: 4 g
- Fat: 7 g
- Sodium: 50 mg
- Potassium: 480 mg
- Phosphorus: 50 mg

Serves: 4 **Cooking Time:** 10 minutes

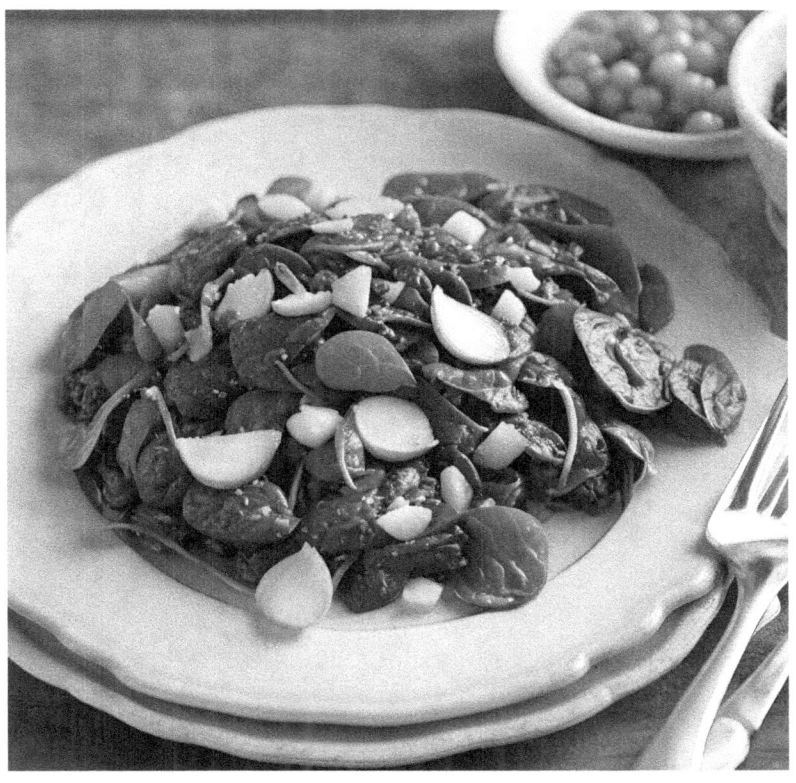

13. Lemon Herb Pasta

Ingredients:
- 12 oz whole wheat spaghetti
- 2 tablespoons olive oil
- Zest and juice of 1 lemon
- 1/4 cup chopped fresh basil
- 1/4 cup chopped fresh parsley
- 2 cloves garlic, minced
- 1/4 cup grated Parmesan cheese (optional)

Instructions:
1. Cook the spaghetti according to package instructions until al dente; drain and set aside.
2. In the same pot, heat olive oil over medium heat.
3. Add garlic and sauté for about 1 minute until fragrant.
4. Add the cooked spaghetti back to the pot along with lemon zest, lemon juice, basil, and parsley.
5. Toss everything together until the pasta is well coated with the lemon-herb mixture.
6. Serve hot, sprinkled with Parmesan cheese if desired.

Nutrition Info Per Serving:
- Calories: 280
- Protein: 10 g
- Carbohydrates: 44 g
- Fat: 7 g
- Sodium: 85 mg
- Potassium: 125 mg
- Phosphorus: 90 mg

Serves: 4 **Cooking Time:** 20 minutes

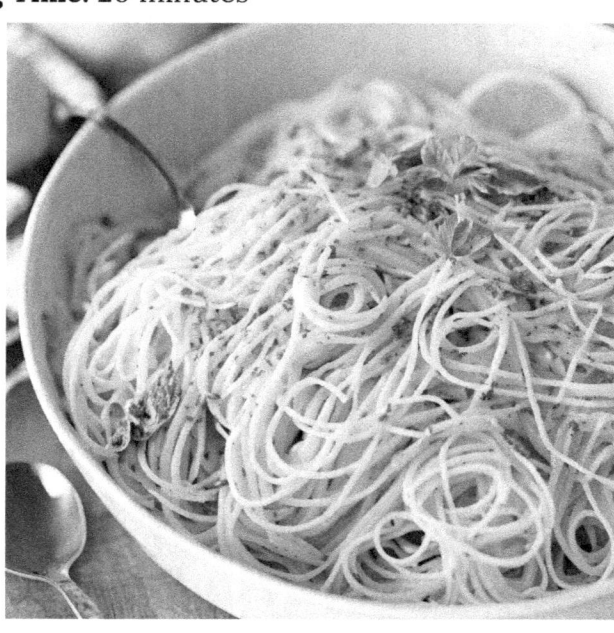

14. Sautéed Mushrooms and Onions

Ingredients:
- 2 cups sliced mushrooms
- 1 large onion, sliced
- 2 tablespoons olive oil
- 1 teaspoon dried thyme

Instructions:
1. Heat olive oil in a large skillet over medium heat.
2. Add the onions and mushrooms to the skillet.
3. Sauté until the onions are translucent and mushrooms are golden, about 8-10 minutes.
4. Sprinkle thyme over the mushrooms and onions and stir to combine.
5. Serve hot.

Nutrition Info Per Serving:
- Calories: 120
- Protein: 2 g
- Carbohydrates: 10 g
- Fat: 8 g
- Sodium: 15 mg
- Potassium: 300 mg
- Phosphorus: 70 mg

Serves: 4 **Cooking Time:** 10 minutes

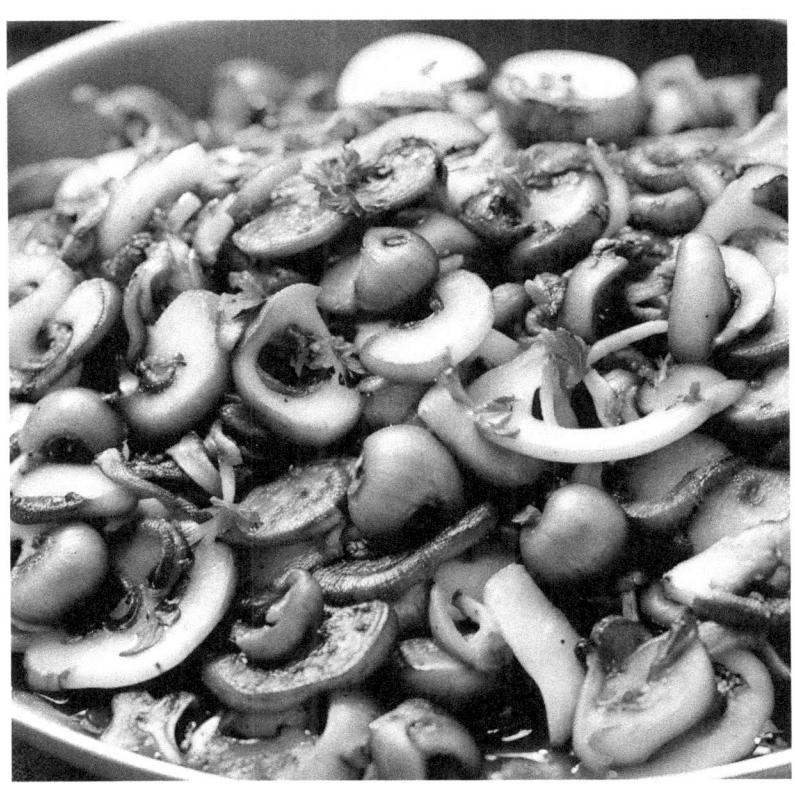

15. Roasted Root Vegetables

Ingredients:
- 2 carrots, peeled and chopped
- 2 parsnips, peeled and chopped
- 1 sweet potato, peeled and chopped
- 2 tablespoons olive oil
- 1 teaspoon dried rosemary

Instructions:
1. Preheat the oven to 400°F (200°C).
2. Place the chopped vegetables on a baking sheet.
3. Drizzle with olive oil and sprinkle with rosemary.
4. Toss to coat evenly.
5. Roast in the oven for 30-35 minutes, stirring occasionally, until vegetables are tender and caramelized.
6. Serve hot.

Nutrition Info Per Serving:
- Calories: 160
- Protein: 2 g
- Carbohydrates: 24 g
- Fat: 7 g
- Sodium: 30 mg
- Potassium: 450 mg
- Phosphorus: 75 mg

Serves: 4 **Cooking Time:** 35 minutes

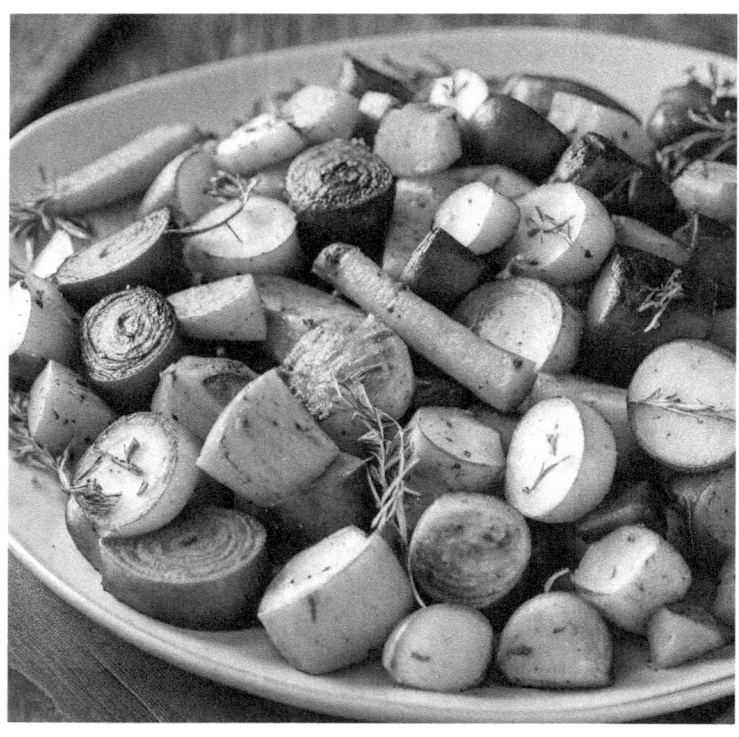

16. Cucumber Gazpacho

Ingredients:
- 2 large cucumbers, peeled and chopped
- 1 green bell pepper, chopped
- 1 onion, chopped
- 2 cloves garlic
- 1/4 cup white wine vinegar
- 1/4 cup olive oil
- 2 cups water
- Fresh herbs (such as dill or parsley), for garnish

Instructions:
1. Combine cucumbers, bell pepper, onion, and garlic in a blender.
2. Add white wine vinegar, olive oil, and water.
3. Blend until smooth.
4. Chill in the refrigerator for at least 2 hours.
5. Serve cold, garnished with fresh herbs.

Nutrition Info Per Serving:
- Calories: 140
- Protein: 1 g
- Carbohydrates: 10 g
- Fat: 11 g
- Sodium: 15 mg
- Potassium: 275 mg
- Phosphorus: 30 mg

Serves: 4 **Preparation Time:** 10 minutes plus chilling time

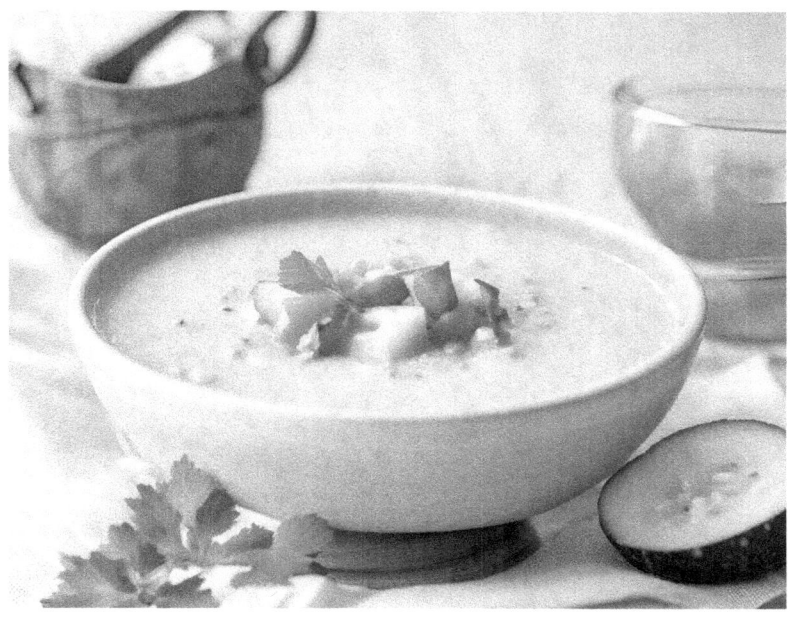

17. Broccoli and Carrot Stir Fry

Ingredients:
- 2 cups broccoli florets
- 1 cup sliced carrots
- 2 tablespoons olive oil
- 1 tablespoon soy sauce (low sodium)
- 1 teaspoon ginger, minced
- 1 clove garlic, minced

Instructions:
1. Heat olive oil in a large skillet over medium heat.
2. Add garlic and ginger, sauté for about 1 minute until fragrant.
3. Add broccoli and carrots to the skillet.
4. Stir-fry for about 5-7 minutes until vegetables are tender yet crisp.
5. Drizzle with soy sauce and toss to coat evenly.
6. Serve hot.

Nutrition Info Per Serving:
- Calories: 120
- Protein: 3 g
- Carbohydrates: 10 g
- Fat: 8 g
- Sodium: 100 mg
- Potassium: 350 mg
- Phosphorus: 45 mg

Serves: 4 **Cooking Time:** 10 minutes

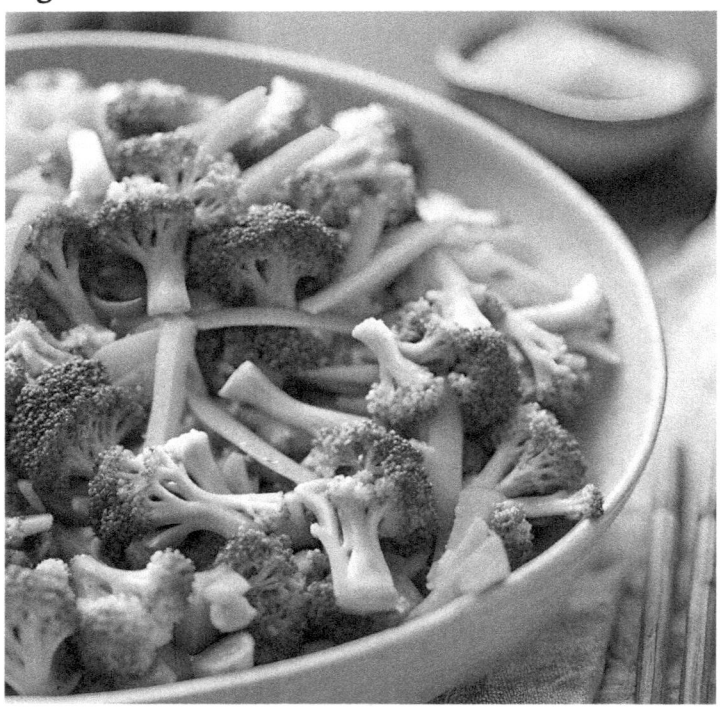

18. Spaghetti Squash with Herbs

Ingredients:
- 1 spaghetti squash, halved lengthwise and seeded
- 2 tablespoons olive oil
- 1/4 cup fresh basil, chopped
- 1/4 cup fresh parsley, chopped
- 2 cloves garlic, minced
- 1 tablespoon lemon juice

Instructions:
1. Preheat oven to 400°F (200°C).
2. Brush the cut sides of the spaghetti squash with olive oil and place cut side down on a baking sheet.
3. Roast in the oven for 40 minutes, or until the flesh is tender and can be shredded with a fork.
4. Remove from oven and let cool slightly. Use a fork to scrape the squash into strands.
5. In a skillet, heat a little olive oil over medium heat. Add garlic and sauté until fragrant.
6. Add the spaghetti squash strands, basil, parsley, and lemon juice. Toss to combine and heat through.
7. Serve warm.

Nutrition Info Per Serving:
- Calories: 150
- Protein: 2 g
- Carbohydrates: 20 g
- Fat: 8 g
- Sodium: 30 mg
- Potassium: 260 mg
- Phosphorus: 55 mg

Serves: 4 **Cooking Time:** 50 minutes

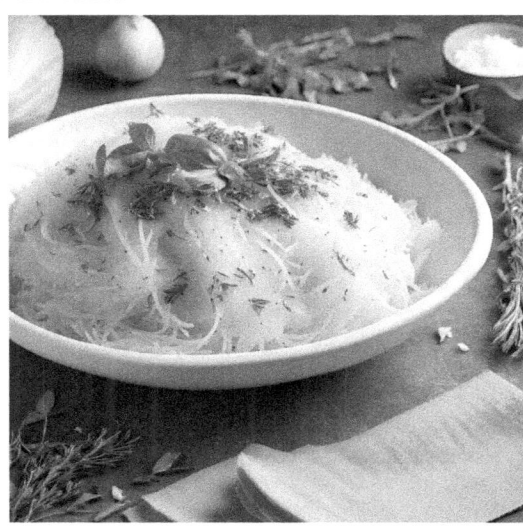

19. Tomato and Basil Bruschetta

Ingredients:
- 1 baguette, sliced into 1/2 inch thick slices
- 4 large tomatoes, diced
- 1/4 cup chopped fresh basil
- 2 cloves garlic, minced
- 2 tablespoons balsamic vinegar
- 2 tablespoons olive oil

Instructions:
1. Preheat oven to 400°F (200°C).
2. Place baguette slices on a baking sheet and toast in the oven for about 5-7 minutes until slightly crispy.
3. In a bowl, combine diced tomatoes, basil, minced garlic, balsamic vinegar, and olive oil.
4. Spoon tomato mixture onto toasted baguette slices.
5. Serve immediately.

Nutrition Info Per Serving:
- Calories: 150
- Protein: 3 g
- Carbohydrates: 20 g
- Fat: 7 g
- Sodium: 180 mg
- Potassium: 210 mg
- Phosphorus: 40 mg

Serves: 6 **Preparation Time:** 20 minutes

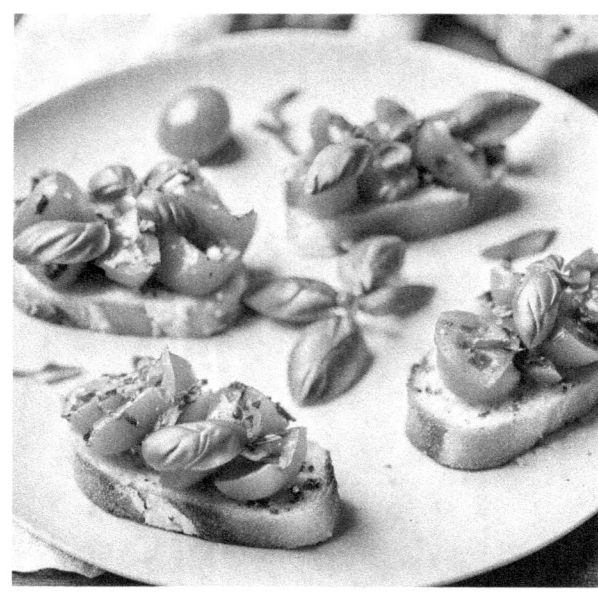

20. Coleslaw with Vinegar Dressing

Ingredients:
- 4 cups shredded cabbage
- 1 carrot, shredded
- 1/4 cup apple cider vinegar
- 2 tablespoons olive oil
- 1 tablespoon honey
- 1 tablespoon Dijon mustard

Instructions:
1. In a large bowl, combine the shredded cabbage and carrot.
2. In a small bowl, whisk together apple cider vinegar, olive oil, honey, and Dijon mustard.
3. Pour the dressing over the cabbage and carrot mixture and toss to coat evenly.
4. Chill in the refrigerator for at least 30 minutes before serving to allow flavors to meld.

Nutrition Info Per Serving:
- Calories: 90
- Protein: 1 g
- Carbohydrates: 10 g
- Fat: 5 g
- Sodium: 45 mg
- Potassium: 120 mg
- Phosphorus: 25 mg

Serves: 4 **Preparation Time:** 40 minutes

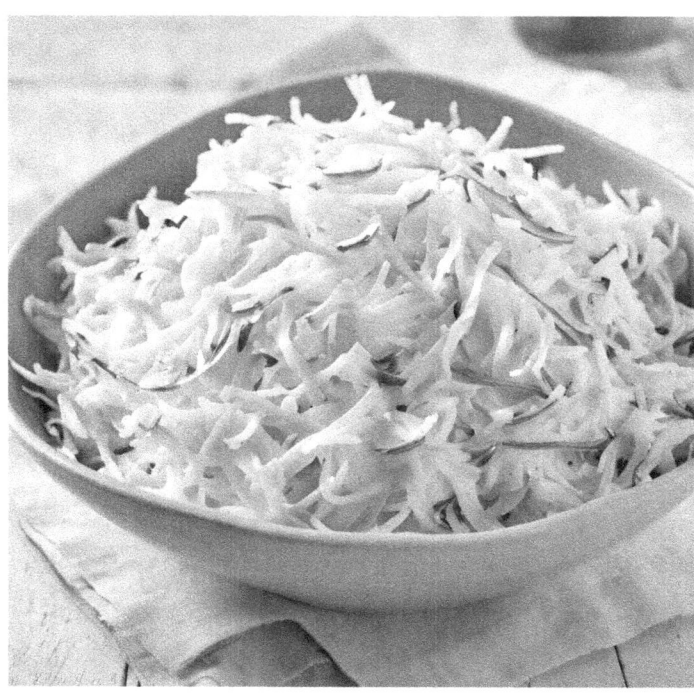

Soups & Salads Recipes

1. Celery Soup
Ingredients:
- 2 tablespoons olive oil
- 1 onion, chopped
- 4 cups chopped celery
- 3 cups low-sodium vegetable broth
- 1/2 cup low-fat milk
- 1 tablespoon fresh lemon juice

Instructions:
1. Heat olive oil in a large pot over medium heat. Add onion and sauté until translucent.
2. Add chopped celery and cook for about 5 minutes, stirring occasionally.
3. Pour in vegetable broth and bring to a boil. Reduce heat and simmer for 20 minutes until celery is soft.
4. Use an immersion blender to puree the soup until smooth.
5. Stir in milk and heat through. Finish with a splash of fresh lemon juice.
6. Serve hot.

Nutrition Info Per Serving:
- Calories: 120
- Protein: 3 g
- Carbohydrates: 14 g
- Fat: 6 g
- Sodium: 100 mg
- Potassium: 360 mg
- Phosphorus: 50 mg

Serves: 4 **Cooking Time:** 30 minutes

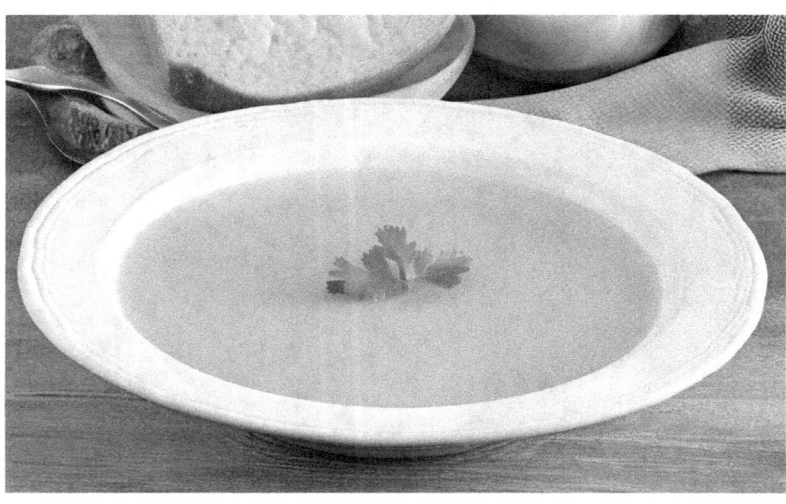

2. Barley Vegetable Soup

Ingredients:
- 1/2 cup pearl barley
- 1 tablespoon olive oil
- 1 onion, diced
- 2 carrots, diced
- 2 celery stalks, diced
- 4 cups low-sodium vegetable broth
- 1 cup diced tomatoes
- 1 cup chopped spinach

Instructions:
1. Rinse barley under cold water.
2. In a large pot, heat olive oil over medium heat. Add onion, carrots, and celery, and sauté until softened.
3. Add barley and vegetable broth. Bring to a boil, then reduce heat and simmer for about 40 minutes, or until barley is tender.
4. Stir in diced tomatoes and spinach, cooking for an additional 5 minutes.
5. Serve hot.

Nutrition Info Per Serving:
- Calories: 180
- Protein: 4 g
- Carbohydrates: 34 g
- Fat: 4 g
- Sodium: 150 mg
- Potassium: 400 mg
- Phosphorus: 95 mg

Serves: 4 **Cooking Time:** 50 minutes

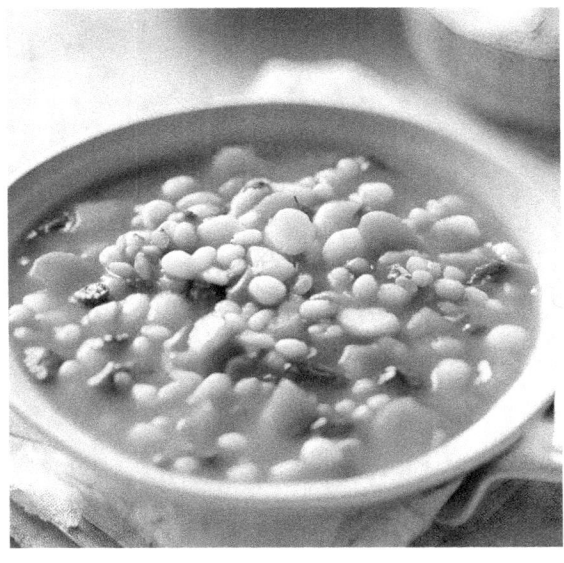

3. Leek and Potato Soup

Ingredients:
- 3 leeks, cleaned and sliced
- 2 large potatoes, peeled and diced
- 1 tablespoon olive oil
- 4 cups low-sodium vegetable broth
- 1/2 cup low-fat milk
- 1 tablespoon chopped fresh parsley

Instructions:
1. In a large pot, heat olive oil over medium heat. Add leeks and sauté until soft.
2. Add diced potatoes and vegetable broth. Bring to a boil, then reduce heat and simmer for 20-25 minutes until potatoes are tender.
3. Puree the soup using an immersion blender until smooth.
4. Stir in milk and warm through. Garnish with fresh parsley before serving.
5. Serve hot.

Nutrition Info Per Serving:
- Calories: 200
- Protein: 5 g
- Carbohydrates: 35 g
- Fat: 5 g
- Sodium: 125 mg
- Potassium: 750 mg
- Phosphorus: 100 mg

Serves: 4 **Cooking Time:** 45 minutes

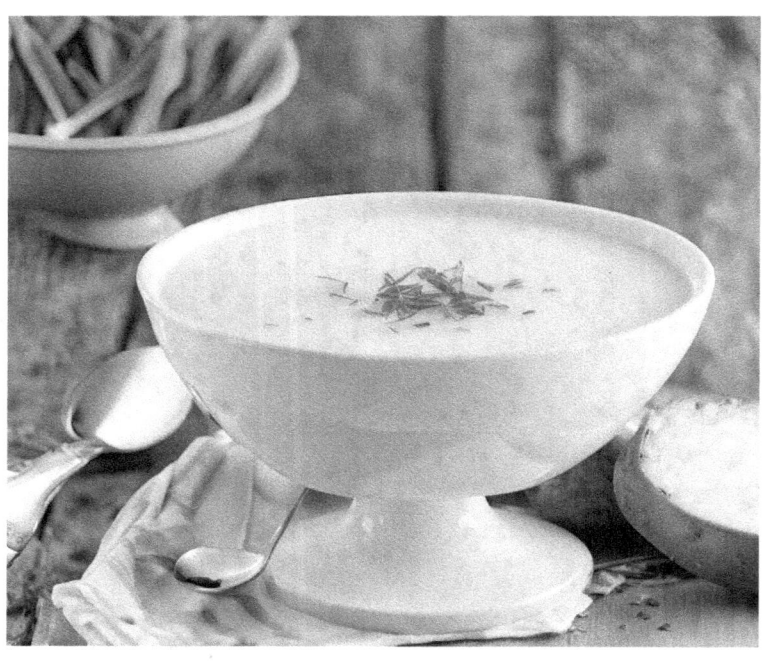

4. Green Bean Soup

Ingredients:
- 4 cups green beans, trimmed and cut into 1-inch pieces
- 1 onion, chopped
- 2 tablespoons olive oil
- 4 cups low-sodium vegetable broth
- 1/2 cup chopped fresh dill

Instructions:
1. In a large pot, heat olive oil over medium heat. Add onion and sauté until translucent.
2. Add green beans and vegetable broth. Bring to a boil, then reduce heat and simmer for 15 minutes, or until beans are tender.
3. Stir in fresh dill and cook for an additional 5 minutes.
4. Serve hot.

Nutrition Info Per Serving:
- Calories: 130
- Protein: 4 g
- Carbohydrates: 18 g
- Fat: 5 g
- Sodium: 100 mg
- Potassium: 340 mg
- Phosphorus: 55 mg

Serves: 4 **Cooking Time:** 25 minutes

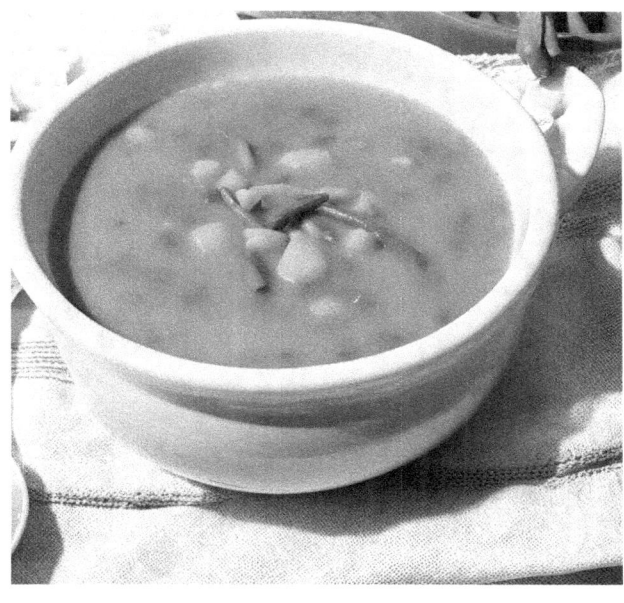

5. Turnip Soup

Ingredients:
- 4 large turnips, peeled and chopped
- 1 onion, chopped
- 2 tablespoons olive oil
- 4 cups low-sodium vegetable broth
- 1/2 cup low-fat milk
- 1 tablespoon fresh thyme, chopped

Instructions:
1. In a large pot, heat olive oil over medium heat. Add onion and sauté until soft.
2. Add chopped turnips and sauté for a few more minutes.
3. Pour in vegetable broth and bring to a boil. Reduce heat and simmer until turnips are tender, about 20 minutes.
4. Use an immersion blender to puree the soup until smooth.
5. Stir in milk and thyme, and heat through.
6. Serve hot.

Nutrition Info Per Serving:
- Calories: 150
- Protein: 3 g
- Carbohydrates: 18 g
- Fat: 7 g
- Sodium: 100 mg
- Potassium: 450 mg
- Phosphorus: 60 mg

Serves: 4 **Cooking Time:** 30 minutes

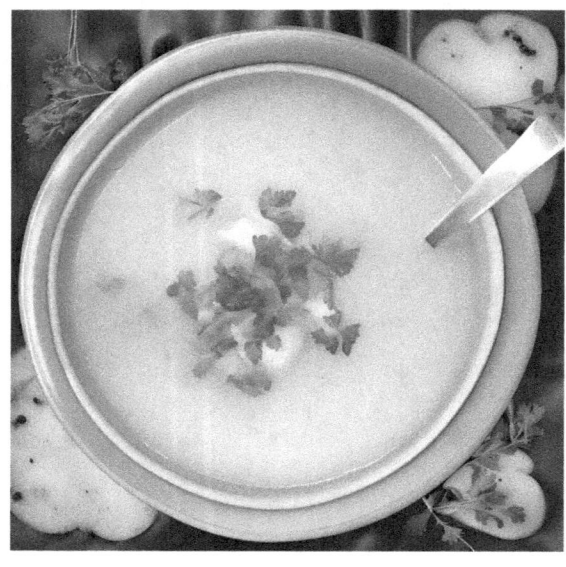

6. Asparagus Soup

Ingredients:
- 2 pounds asparagus, trimmed and chopped
- 1 onion, chopped
- 2 cloves garlic, minced
- 2 tablespoons olive oil
- 4 cups low-sodium vegetable broth
- 1/2 cup low-fat cream

Instructions:
1. In a large pot, heat olive oil over medium heat. Add onion and garlic, and sauté until onion is translucent.
2. Add chopped asparagus and cook for a few minutes.
3. Pour in vegetable broth and bring to a boil. Reduce heat and simmer until asparagus is very tender, about 15 minutes.
4. Puree the mixture with an immersion blender until smooth.
5. Stir in cream and warm the soup just before serving.
6. Serve hot.

Nutrition Info Per Serving:
- Calories: 180
- Protein: 6 g
- Carbohydrates: 15 g
- Fat: 11 g
- Sodium: 75 mg
- Potassium: 490 mg
- Phosphorus: 95 mg

Serves: 4 **Cooking Time:** 30 minutes

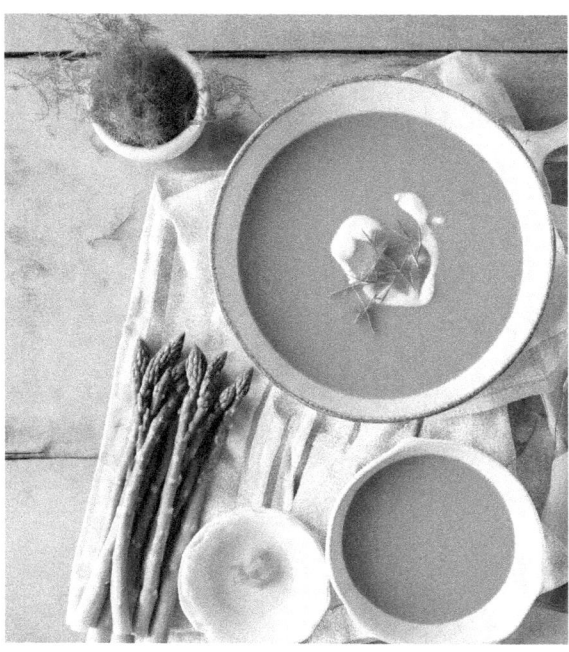

7. Squash and Apple Soup

Ingredients:
- 1 butternut squash, peeled, seeded, and chopped
- 2 apples, peeled and chopped
- 1 onion, chopped
- 2 tablespoons olive oil
- 4 cups low-sodium vegetable broth
- 1 teaspoon ground cinnamon

Instructions:
1. In a large pot, heat olive oil over medium heat. Add onion and sauté until soft.
2. Add squash and apples, and cook for a few minutes.
3. Add vegetable broth and cinnamon. Bring to a boil, then reduce heat and simmer until squash and apples are tender, about 25 minutes.
4. Puree the soup with an immersion blender until smooth.
5. Serve hot.

Nutrition Info Per Serving:
- Calories: 190
- Protein: 2 g
- Carbohydrates: 35 g
- Fat: 5 g
- Sodium: 75 mg
- Potassium: 500 mg
- Phosphorus: 70 mg

Serves: 4 **Cooking Time:** 40 minutes

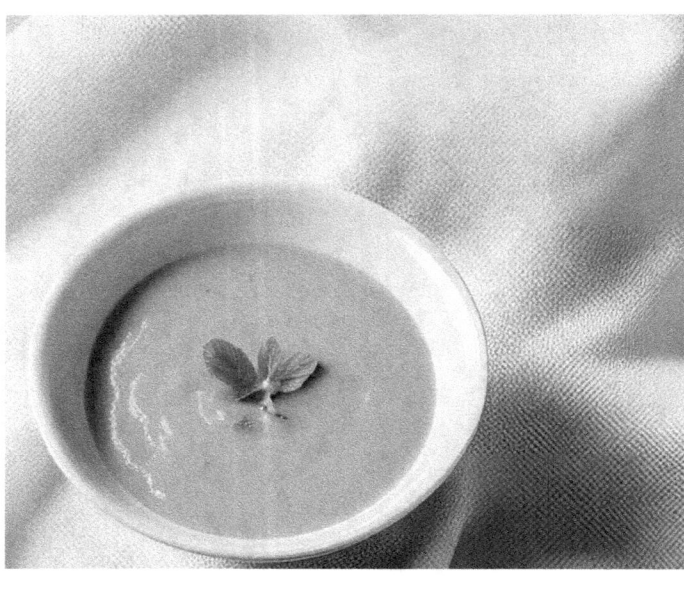

8. Cucumber Dill Soup

Ingredients:
- 2 large cucumbers, peeled, seeded, and chopped
- 1/4 cup fresh dill, chopped
- 2 cups plain low-fat yogurt
- 1 clove garlic, minced
- 2 tablespoons lemon juice
- 1 tablespoon olive oil

Instructions:
1. In a blender, combine cucumbers, dill, yogurt, garlic, and lemon juice.
2. Blend until smooth.
3. Chill in the refrigerator for at least 2 hours.
4. Drizzle with olive oil before serving.
5. Serve cold.

Nutrition Info Per Serving:
- Calories: 150
- Protein: 6 g
- Carbohydrates: 16 g
- Fat: 7 g
- Sodium: 50 mg
- Potassium: 440 mg
- Phosphorus: 140 mg

Serves: 4 **Preparation Time:** 10 minutes plus chilling time

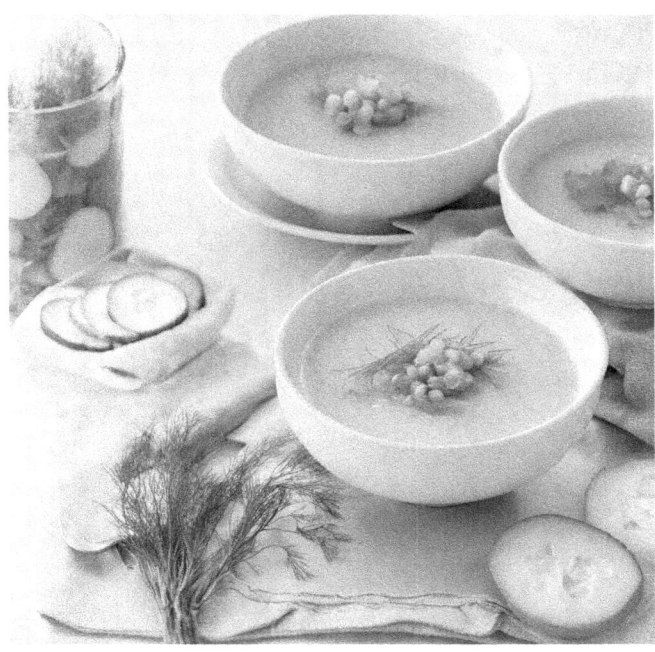

9. Parsnip Soup

Ingredients:
- 4 parsnips, peeled and chopped
- 1 onion, chopped
- 2 tablespoons olive oil
- 4 cups low-sodium vegetable broth
- 1/2 cup low-fat milk
- 1 teaspoon dried thyme

Instructions:
1. In a large pot, heat olive oil over medium heat. Add onion and sauté until translucent.
2. Add chopped parsnips and cook for a few minutes.
3. Pour in vegetable broth and bring to a boil. Reduce heat and simmer until parsnips are tender, about 20 minutes.
4. Puree the soup using an immersion blender until smooth.
5. Stir in milk and thyme, and warm the soup through.
6. Serve hot.

Nutrition Info Per Serving:
- Calories: 180
- Protein: 3 g
- Carbohydrates: 27 g
- Fat: 7 g
- Sodium: 100 mg
- Potassium: 450 mg
- Phosphorus: 70 mg

Serves: 4 **Cooking Time:** 30 minutes

10. Red Bell Pepper Soup

Ingredients:
- 4 red bell peppers, seeded and chopped
- 1 onion, chopped
- 2 cloves garlic, minced
- 2 tablespoons olive oil
- 4 cups low-sodium vegetable broth
- 1/2 cup low-fat cream

Instructions:
1. In a large pot, heat olive oil over medium heat. Add onion and garlic, and sauté until onion is soft.
2. Add chopped bell peppers and cook for a few minutes.
3. Add vegetable broth and bring to a boil. Reduce heat and simmer until bell peppers are very tender, about 20 minutes.
4. Puree the soup with an immersion blender until smooth.
5. Stir in cream and gently reheat.
6. Serve hot.

Nutrition Info Per Serving:
- Calories: 190
- Protein: 3 g
- Carbohydrates: 18 g
- Fat: 12 g
- Sodium: 80 mg
- Potassium: 250 mg
- Phosphorus: 60 mg

Serves: 4 **Cooking Time:** 30 minutes

11. Iceberg Lettuce with Radishes

Ingredients:
- 1 head iceberg lettuce, chopped
- 1 cup radishes, thinly sliced
- 2 tablespoons olive oil
- 2 tablespoons white wine vinegar
- 1 tablespoon honey

Instructions:
1. In a large salad bowl, combine chopped lettuce and sliced radishes.
2. In a small bowl, whisk together olive oil, white wine vinegar, and honey.
3. Drizzle the dressing over the salad and toss to coat evenly.
4. Serve immediately.

Nutrition Info Per Serving:
- Calories: 110
- Protein: 1 g
- Carbohydrates: 8 g
- Fat: 8 g
- Sodium: 50 mg
- Potassium: 270 mg
- Phosphorus: 30 mg

Serves: 4 **Preparation Time:** 10 minutes

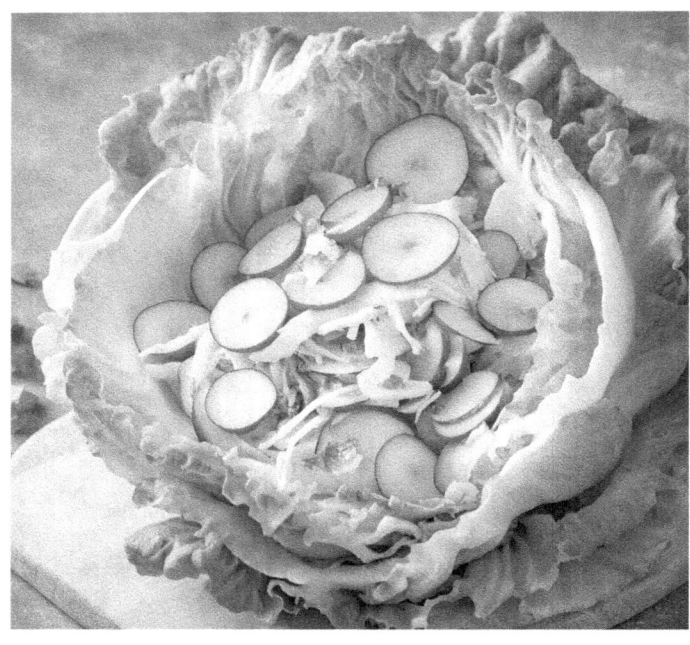

12. Shredded Beet and Carrot Salad

Ingredients:
- 2 large beets, peeled and shredded
- 2 large carrots, peeled and shredded
- 2 tablespoons olive oil
- 2 tablespoons lemon juice
- 1 tablespoon chopped fresh parsley

Instructions:
1. In a large salad bowl, combine shredded beets and carrots.
2. In a small bowl, whisk together olive oil and lemon juice.
3. Pour the dressing over the salad and toss to coat evenly.
4. Garnish with fresh parsley before serving.
5. Serve chilled or at room temperature.

Nutrition Info Per Serving:
- Calories: 150
- Protein: 2 g
- Carbohydrates: 18 g
- Fat: 8 g
- Sodium: 85 mg
- Potassium: 360 mg
- Phosphorus: 50 mg

Serves: 4 **Preparation Time:** 15 minutes

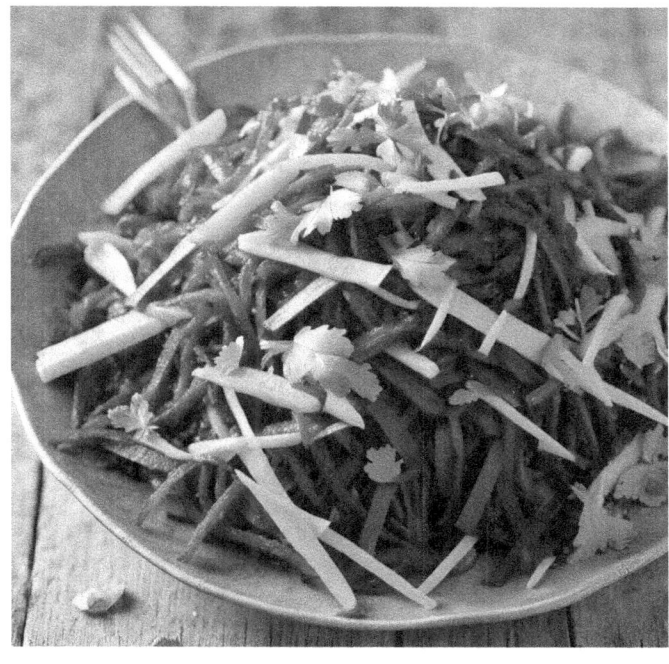

13. Borscht (Beet Soup)

Ingredients:
- 4 medium beets, peeled and diced
- 2 carrots, peeled and diced
- 1 onion, chopped
- 2 potatoes, peeled and diced
- 1/2 head cabbage, shredded
- 6 cups low-sodium vegetable broth
- 2 tablespoons apple cider vinegar
- 1 tablespoon honey
- 1/2 cup sour cream (for garnish)
- Fresh dill (for garnish)

Instructions:
1. In a large pot, combine beets, carrots, onion, potatoes, and vegetable broth. Bring to a boil.
2. Reduce heat to a simmer and cook until vegetables are tender, about 30 minutes.
3. Add shredded cabbage and cook for an additional 10 minutes.
4. Stir in apple cider vinegar and honey.
5. Serve hot, topped with a dollop of sour cream and a sprinkle of fresh dill.

Nutrition Info Per Serving:
- Calories: 180
- Protein: 4 g
- Carbohydrates: 30 g
- Fat: 5 g
- Sodium: 150 mg
- Potassium: 850 mg
- Phosphorus: 70 mg

Serves: 6 **Cooking Time:** 45 minutes

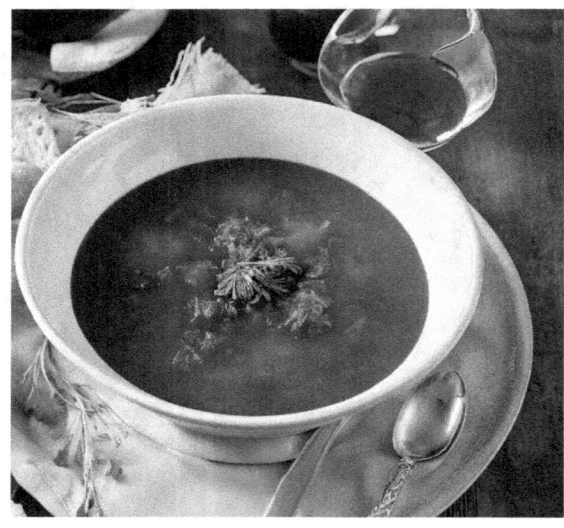

14. Chilled Asparagus Salad

Ingredients:
- 1 pound asparagus, trimmed and blanched
- 1/4 cup sliced almonds, toasted
- 2 tablespoons olive oil
- 2 tablespoons lemon juice
- 1 teaspoon grated lemon zest

Instructions:
1. Cut the blanched asparagus into 1-inch pieces.
2. In a salad bowl, combine asparagus, sliced almonds, olive oil, lemon juice, and lemon zest.
3. Toss gently to combine.
4. Chill in the refrigerator for at least 30 minutes before serving.

Nutrition Info Per Serving:
- Calories: 120
- Protein: 4 g
- Carbohydrates: 6 g
- Fat: 10 g
- Sodium: 30 mg
- Potassium: 230 mg
- Phosphorus: 50 mg

Serves: 4 **Preparation Time:** 40 minutes

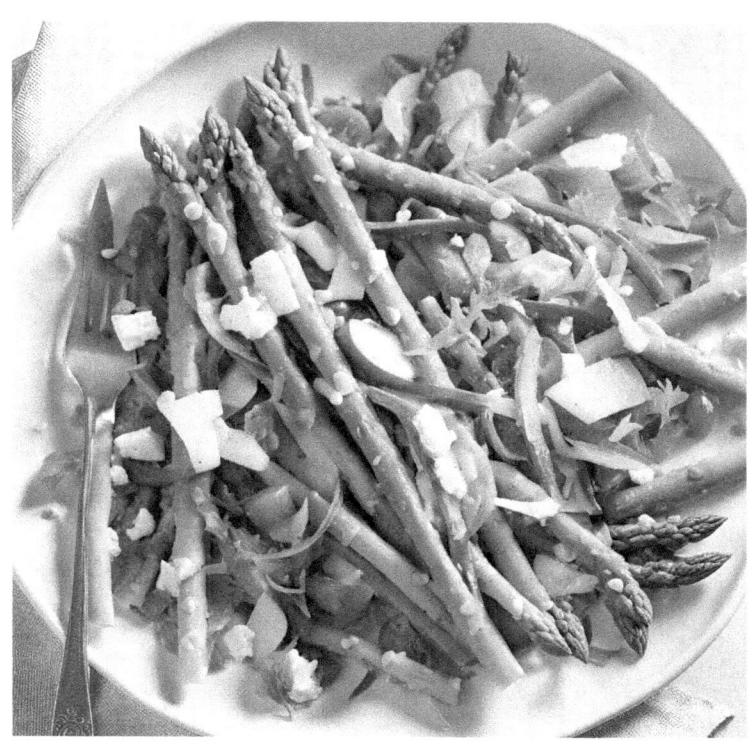

15. Roasted Bell Pepper Salad

Ingredients:
- 4 bell peppers (varied colors), roasted and peeled
- 2 tablespoons capers
- 1/4 cup olive oil
- 2 tablespoons balsamic vinegar
- Fresh basil leaves, chopped

Instructions:
1. Slice the roasted bell peppers into strips.
2. In a salad bowl, combine bell pepper strips, capers, olive oil, balsamic vinegar, and chopped basil.
3. Toss to combine.
4. Serve at room temperature or chilled.

Nutrition Info Per Serving:
- Calories: 150
- Protein: 1 g
- Carbohydrates: 10 g
- Fat: 12 g
- Sodium: 80 mg
- Potassium: 250 mg
- Phosphorus: 20 mg

Serves: 4 **Preparation Time:** 20 minutes (plus time for roasting)

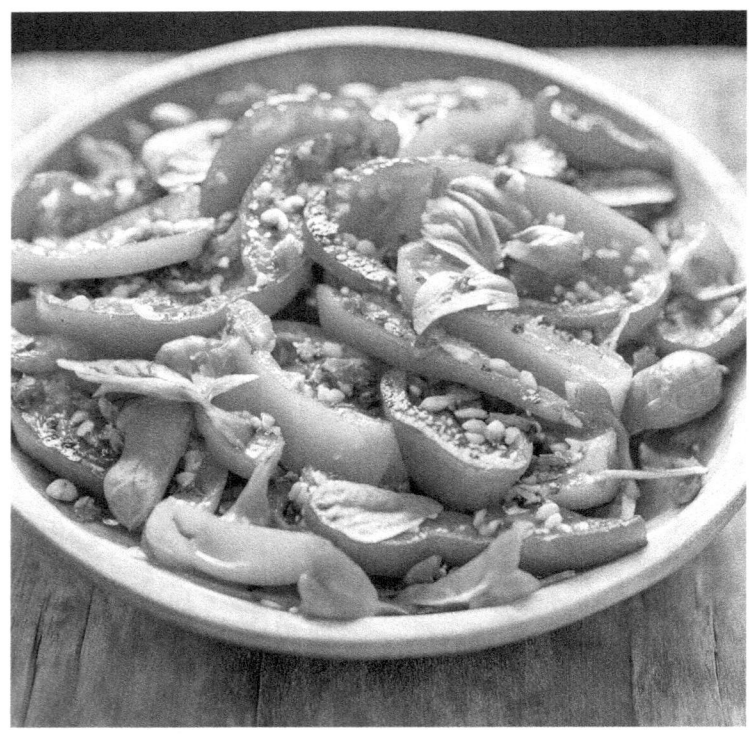

16. Tomato and Cucumber Gazpacho Salad

Ingredients:
- 3 tomatoes, diced
- 1 cucumber, peeled and diced
- 1 red bell pepper, diced
- 1 onion, chopped
- 2 cloves garlic, minced
- 1/4 cup olive oil
- 2 tablespoons red wine vinegar
- 1 cup tomato juice

Instructions:
1. In a large bowl, combine tomatoes, cucumber, bell pepper, onion, and garlic.
2. In a small bowl, whisk together olive oil, red wine vinegar, and tomato juice.
3. Pour the dressing over the vegetables and toss to coat.
4. Chill in the refrigerator for at least 2 hours before serving to allow flavors to meld.

Nutrition Info Per Serving:
- Calories: 180
- Protein: 2 g
- Carbohydrates: 15 g
- Fat: 13 g
- Sodium: 55 mg
- Potassium: 420 mg
- Phosphorus: 45 mg

Serves: 4 **Preparation Time:** 15 minutes plus chilling

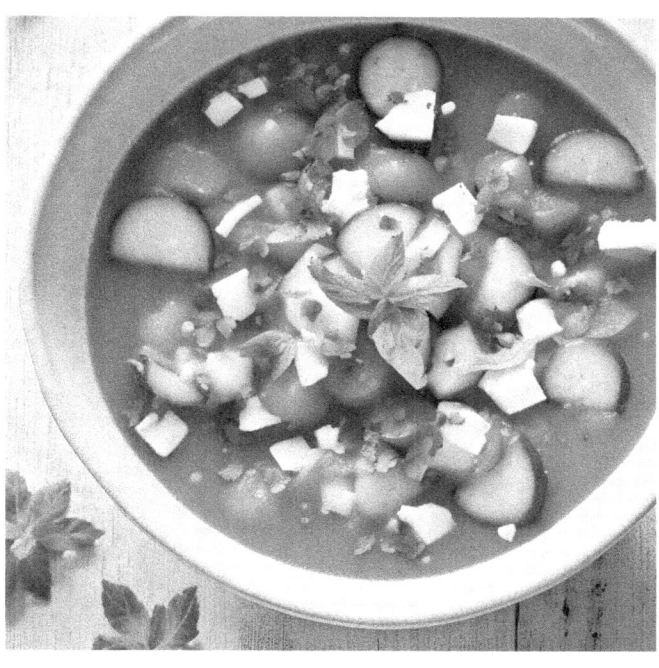

17. Endive and Pear Salad

Ingredients:
- 3 endives, leaves separated and washed
- 2 ripe pears, cored and sliced
- 1/4 cup walnuts, toasted and chopped
- 1/4 cup crumbled feta cheese
- 2 tablespoons olive oil
- 1 tablespoon apple cider vinegar
- 1 teaspoon honey

Instructions:
1. Arrange endive leaves in a large salad bowl.
2. Top with sliced pears, toasted walnuts, and crumbled feta cheese.
3. In a small bowl, whisk together olive oil, apple cider vinegar, and honey.
4. Drizzle the dressing over the salad.
5. Serve immediately.

Nutrition Info Per Serving:
- Calories: 180
- Protein: 4 g
- Carbohydrates: 14 g
- Fat: 12 g
- Sodium: 125 mg
- Potassium: 350 mg
- Phosphorus: 50 mg

Serves: 4 **Preparation Time:** 15 minutes

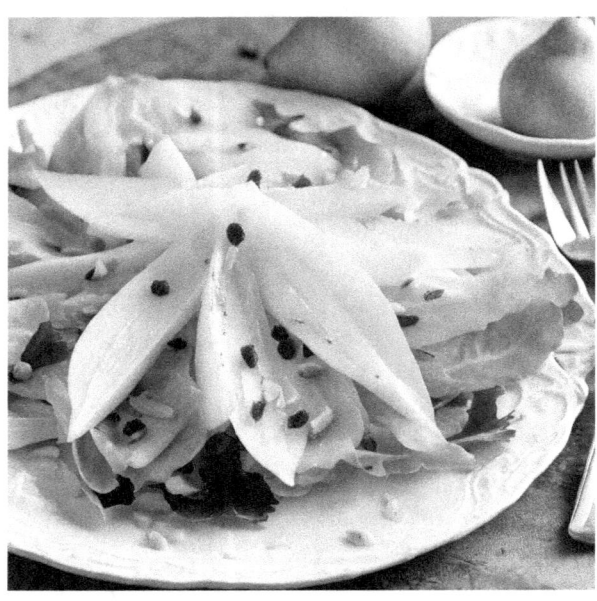

18. Jicama Salad

Ingredients:
- 1 large jicama, peeled and julienned
- 1 carrot, peeled and julienned
- 1 red bell pepper, julienned
- 1/4 cup fresh lime juice
- 1 tablespoon olive oil
- 1/4 cup chopped fresh cilantro

Instructions:
1. In a large bowl, combine jicama, carrot, and red bell pepper.
2. In a small bowl, whisk together lime juice and olive oil.
3. Pour the dressing over the vegetables and toss to coat evenly.
4. Stir in chopped cilantro.
5. Chill in the refrigerator for about 30 minutes before serving to allow flavors to meld.

Nutrition Info Per Serving:
- Calories: 100
- Protein: 1 g
- Carbohydrates: 16 g
- Fat: 4 g
- Sodium: 20 mg
- Potassium: 270 mg
- Phosphorus: 35 mg

Serves: 4 **Preparation Time:** 40 minutes

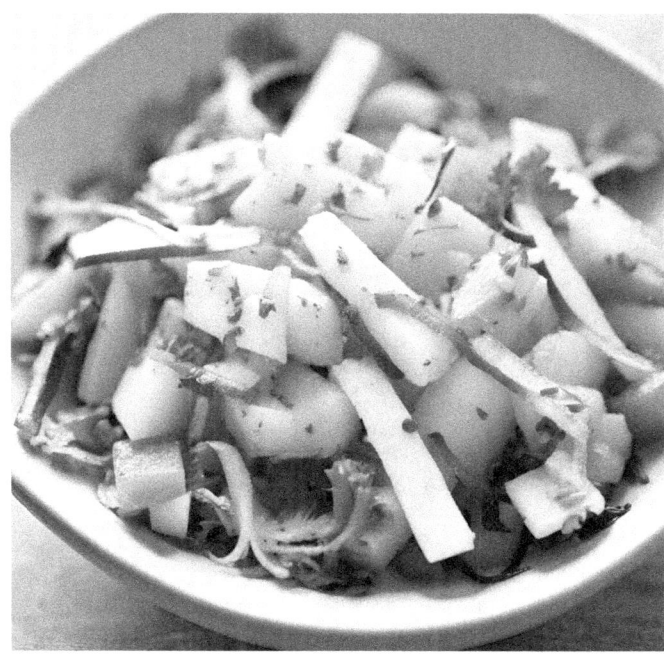

19. Radish and Green Onion Salad

Ingredients:
- 2 cups sliced radishes
- 1 cup chopped green onions
- 2 tablespoons olive oil
- 2 tablespoons lemon juice
- 1 teaspoon grated ginger

Instructions:
1. In a salad bowl, combine sliced radishes and chopped green onions.
2. In a small bowl, whisk together olive oil, lemon juice, and grated ginger.
3. Drizzle the dressing over the radish and green onion mixture.
4. Toss to combine.
5. Serve chilled or at room temperature.

Nutrition Info Per Serving:
- Calories: 100
- Protein: 1 g
- Carbohydrates: 6 g
- Fat: 8 g
- Sodium: 30 mg
- Potassium: 270 mg
- Phosphorus: 30 mg

Serves: 4 **Preparation Time:** 10 minutes

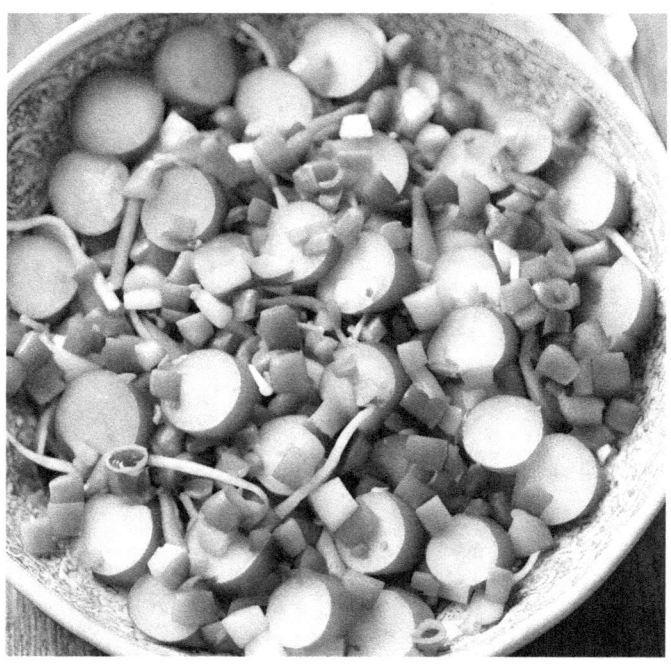

20. Mixed Greens with Apple Slices

Ingredients:
- 4 cups mixed greens (such as spinach, arugula, and lettuce)
- 1 apple, cored and thinly sliced
- 1/4 cup dried cranberries
- 1/4 cup pecans, toasted
- 2 tablespoons balsamic vinegar
- 2 tablespoons olive oil

Instructions:
1. In a large salad bowl, combine mixed greens, sliced apple, dried cranberries, and toasted pecans.
2. In a small bowl, whisk together balsamic vinegar and olive oil.
3. Drizzle the dressing over the salad and toss gently to combine.
4. Serve immediately.

Nutrition Info Per Serving:
- Calories: 180
- Protein: 2 g
- Carbohydrates: 18 g
- Fat: 12 g
- Sodium: 30 mg
- Potassium: 300 mg
- Phosphorus: 50 mg

Serves: 4 **Preparation Time:** 10 minutes

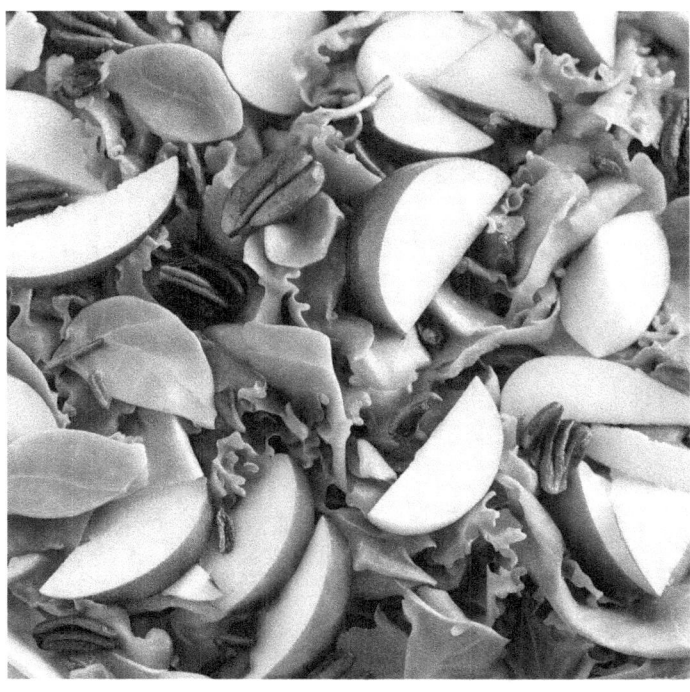

Snacks and Sides

1. Apple Chips

Ingredients:
- 2 apples (such as Granny Smith or Fuji)
- 1 teaspoon cinnamon

Instructions:
1. Preheat your oven to 200°F (95°C).
2. Core the apples and slice them thinly.
3. Arrange apple slices in a single layer on a baking sheet lined with parchment paper.
4. Sprinkle cinnamon evenly over the apple slices.
5. Bake for 1 to 2 hours, flipping the slices halfway through, until the apple slices are dried out but still pliable.
6. Cool completely on a wire rack before serving.

Nutrition Info Per Serving:
- Calories: 50
- Protein: 0 g
- Carbohydrates: 13 g
- Fat: 0 g
- Sodium: 0 mg
- Potassium: 100 mg
- Phosphorus: 10 mg

Serves: 4 **Cooking Time:** 2 hours

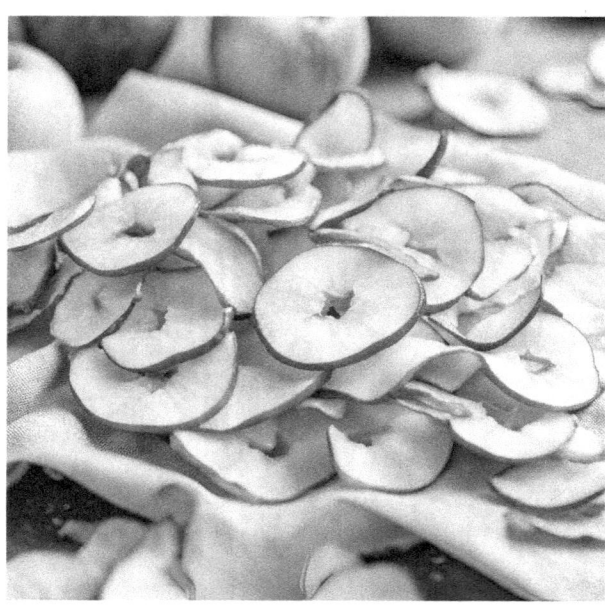

2. Rice Cakes with Unsweetened Apple Sauce

Ingredients:
- 4 plain rice cakes
- 1 cup unsweetened apple sauce

Instructions:
1. Spread approximately 1/4 cup of unsweetened apple sauce over each rice cake.
2. Serve immediately for best texture.

Nutrition Info Per Serving:
- Calories: 70
- Protein: 1 g
- Carbohydrates: 15 g
- Fat: 0 g
- Sodium: 10 mg
- Potassium: 50 mg
- Phosphorus: 10 mg

Serves: 4 **Preparation Time:** 5 minutes

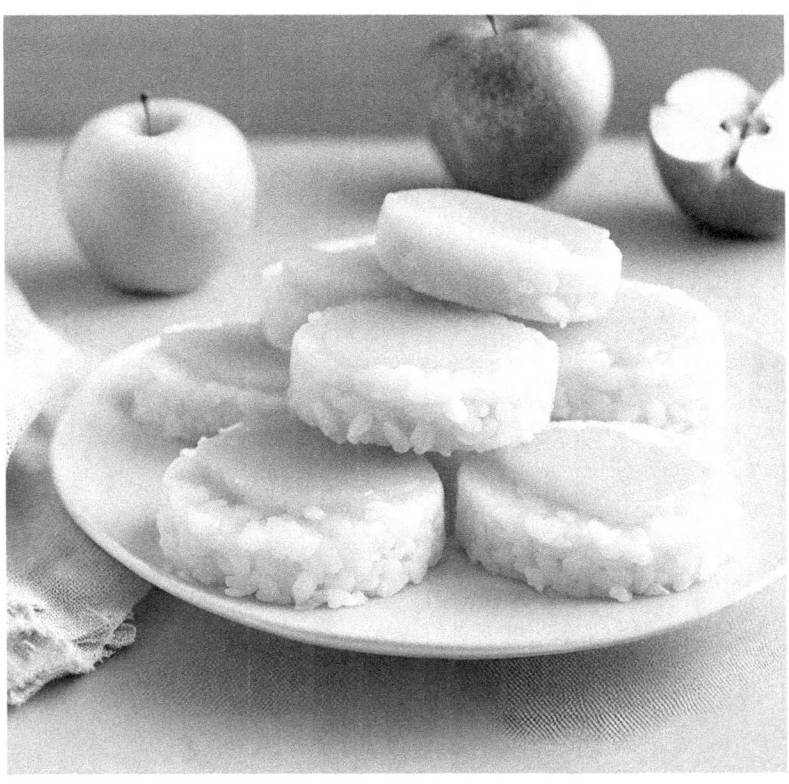

3. Homemade Popcorn

Ingredients:
- 1/4 cup popcorn kernels
- 1 tablespoon olive oil

Instructions:
1. In a large pot with a lid, heat the olive oil over medium heat.
2. Add the popcorn kernels and cover with a lid.
3. Once the kernels start popping, shake the pot occasionally until the popping slows down to several seconds between pops.
4. Remove from heat and transfer to a serving bowl.

Nutrition Info Per Serving:
- Calories: 100
- Protein: 2 g
- Carbohydrates: 12 g
- Fat: 5 g
- Sodium: 0 mg
- Potassium: 30 mg
- Phosphorus: 40 mg

Serves: 4 **Cooking Time:** 10 minutes

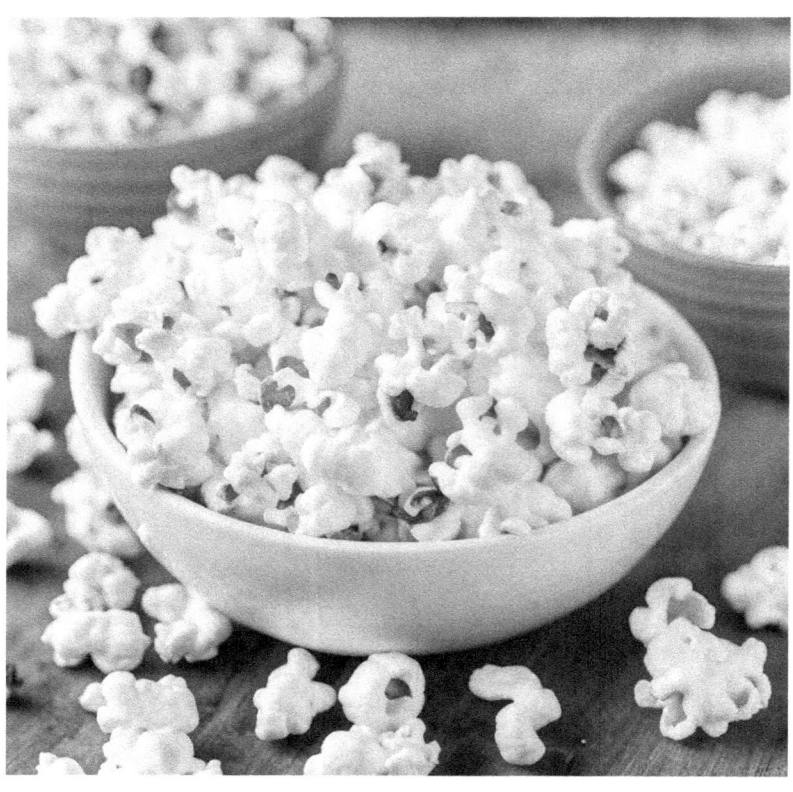

4. Cucumber and Dill Bites

Ingredients:
- 1 large cucumber, sliced into rounds
- 1/4 cup cream cheese (low fat)
- 1 tablespoon fresh dill, chopped

Instructions:
1. Spread a small amount of cream cheese on each cucumber round.
2. Sprinkle fresh dill over the cream cheese.
3. Serve immediately or chill until serving.

Nutrition Info Per Serving:
- Calories: 25
- Protein: 1 g
- Carbohydrates: 2 g
- Fat: 2 g
- Sodium: 20 mg
- Potassium: 45 mg
- Phosphorus: 10 mg

Serves: 4 **Preparation Time:** 10 minutes

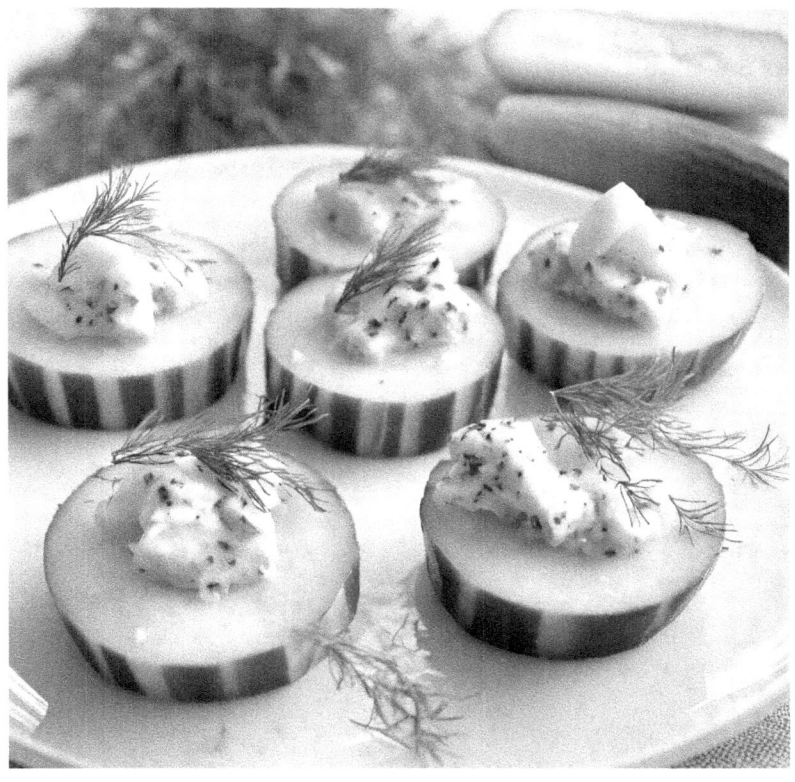

5. Garlic Toast

Ingredients:
- 4 slices of whole wheat bread
- 2 cloves garlic, minced
- 2 tablespoons olive oil

Instructions:
1. Preheat your oven to 400°F (200°C).
2. In a small bowl, combine olive oil and minced garlic.
3. Brush the garlic oil mixture over each slice of bread.
4. Place the bread on a baking sheet and toast in the oven for about 5-10 minutes, or until crispy and golden.
5. Serve warm.

Nutrition Info Per Serving:
- Calories: 140
- Protein: 3 g
- Carbohydrates: 18 g
- Fat: 7 g
- Sodium: 120 mg
- Potassium: 70 mg
- Phosphorus: 40 mg

Serves: 4 **Cooking Time:** 15 minutes

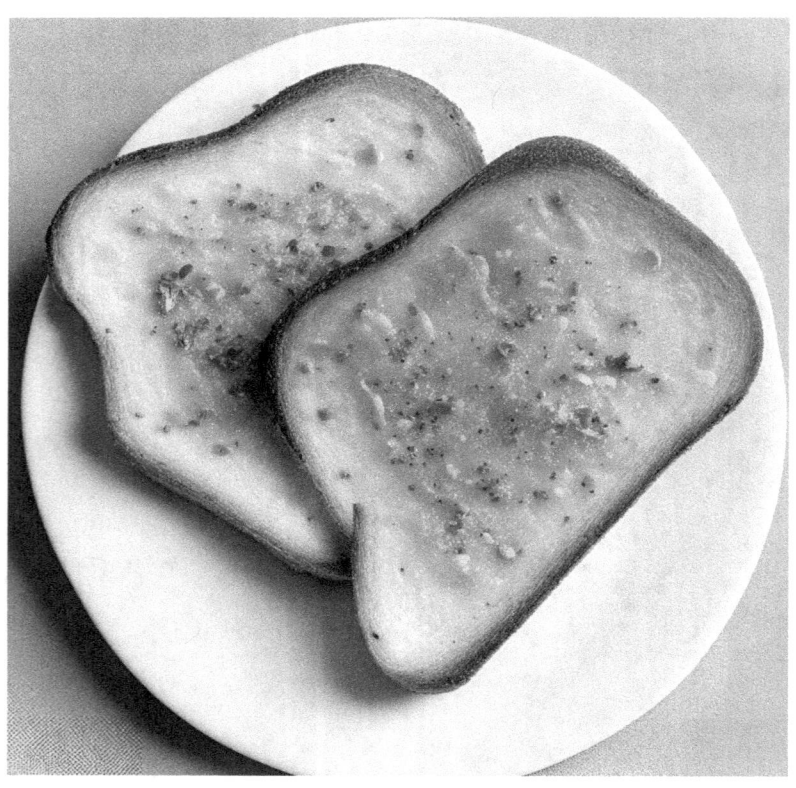

6. Baked Parsnip Fries

Ingredients:
- 4 large parsnips, peeled and cut into fries
- 2 tablespoons olive oil
- 1 teaspoon paprika

Instructions:
1. Preheat oven to 400°F (200°C).
2. Toss the parsnip fries with olive oil and paprika.
3. Spread on a baking sheet in a single layer.
4. Bake for 25-30 minutes, turning halfway through, until golden and crispy.
5. Serve hot.

Nutrition Info Per Serving:
- Calories: 140
- Protein: 2 g
- Carbohydrates: 24 g
- Fat: 5 g
- Sodium: 20 mg
- Potassium: 450 mg
- Phosphorus: 75 mg

Serves: 4 **Cooking Time:** 30 minutes

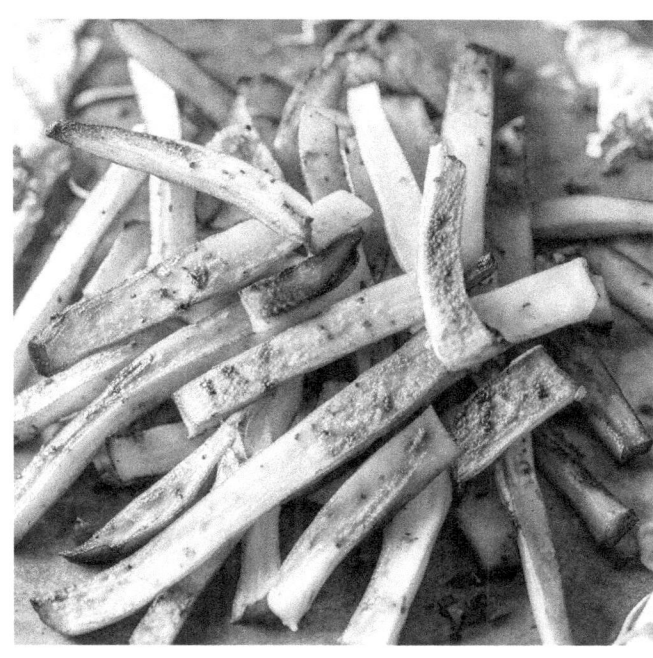

7. Zucchini Chips

Ingredients:
- 2 large zucchinis, thinly sliced
- 1 tablespoon olive oil
- 1 teaspoon dried oregano

Instructions:
1. Preheat oven to 225°F (105°C).
2. Toss zucchini slices with olive oil and oregano.
3. Place in a single layer on a baking sheet lined with parchment paper.
4. Bake for 1.5-2 hours, flipping the slices halfway through, until crisp and golden.
5. Serve cool.

Nutrition Info Per Serving:
- Calories: 50
- Protein: 2 g
- Carbohydrates: 4 g
- Fat: 4 g
- Sodium: 10 mg
- Potassium: 295 mg
- Phosphorus: 30 mg

Serves: 4 **Cooking Time:** Up to 2 hours

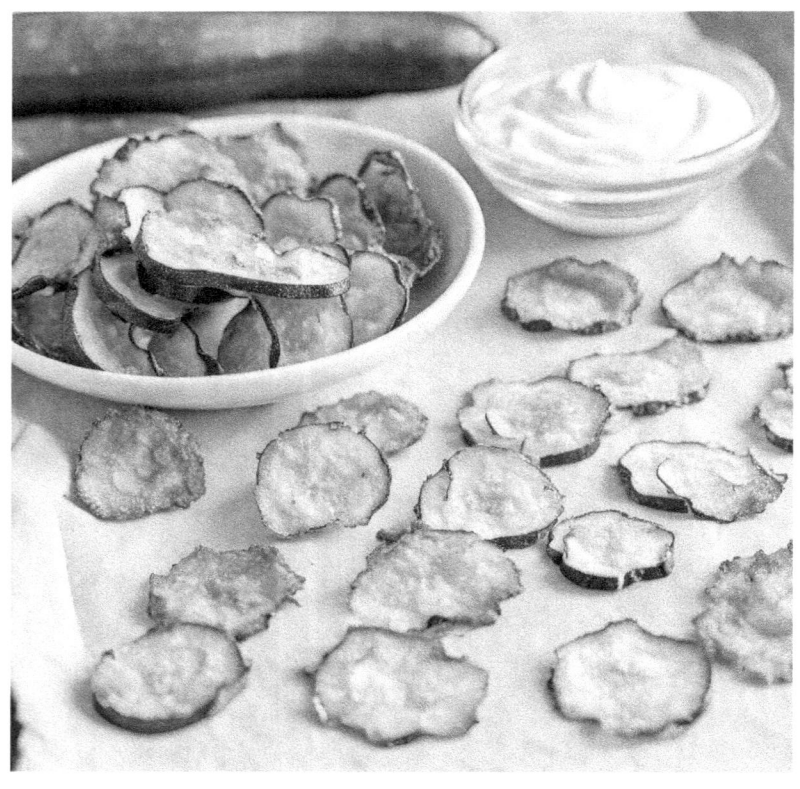

8. Carrot Sticks with Homemade Tzatziki

Ingredients:
- 4 large carrots, peeled and cut into sticks
- 1 cup Greek yogurt
- 1/2 cucumber, grated and drained
- 2 cloves garlic, minced
- 1 tablespoon lemon juice
- 1 tablespoon fresh dill, chopped

Instructions:
1. In a bowl, combine Greek yogurt, grated cucumber, minced garlic, lemon juice, and dill. Mix well to create tzatziki.
2. Chill the tzatziki in the refrigerator.
3. Serve carrot sticks alongside chilled tzatziki for dipping.

Nutrition Info Per Serving:
- Calories: 100
- Protein: 6 g
- Carbohydrates: 12 g
- Fat: 3 g
- Sodium: 50 mg
- Potassium: 360 mg
- Phosphorus: 100 mg

Serves: 4 **Preparation Time:** 15 minutes

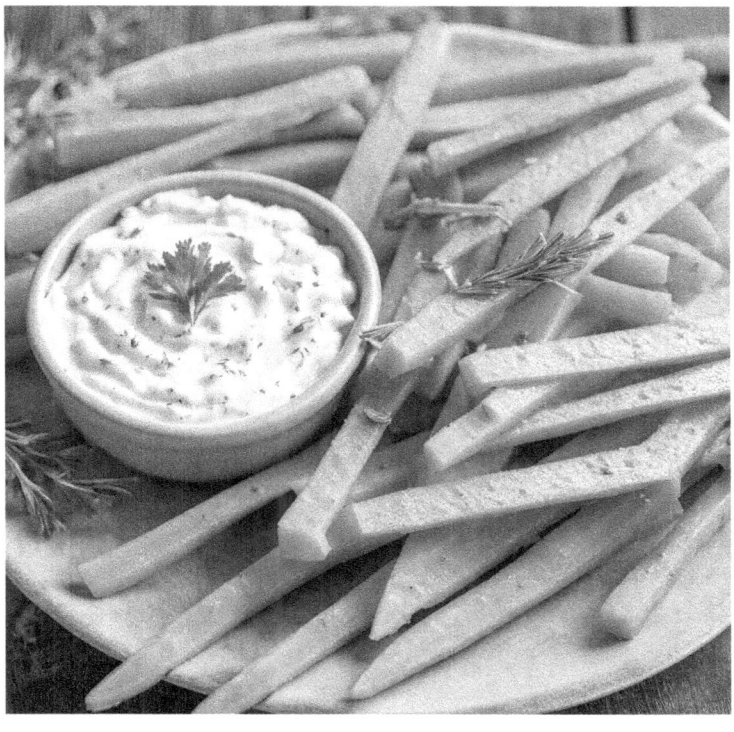

9. Puffed Rice Bars

Ingredients:
- 2 cups puffed rice cereal
- 1/2 cup honey
- 1/2 cup peanut butter

Instructions:
1. In a saucepan, heat honey and peanut butter over medium heat until melted and combined.
2. Remove from heat and stir in puffed rice until well coated.
3. Press the mixture into a greased 8x8 inch pan.
4. Let set in the refrigerator until firm, about 1 hour.
5. Cut into bars and serve.

Nutrition Info Per Serving:
- Calories: 180
- Protein: 4 g
- Carbohydrates: 28 g
- Fat: 7 g
- Sodium: 80 mg
- Potassium: 90 mg
- Phosphorus: 75 mg

Serves: 8 **Preparation Time:** 1 hour 10 minutes

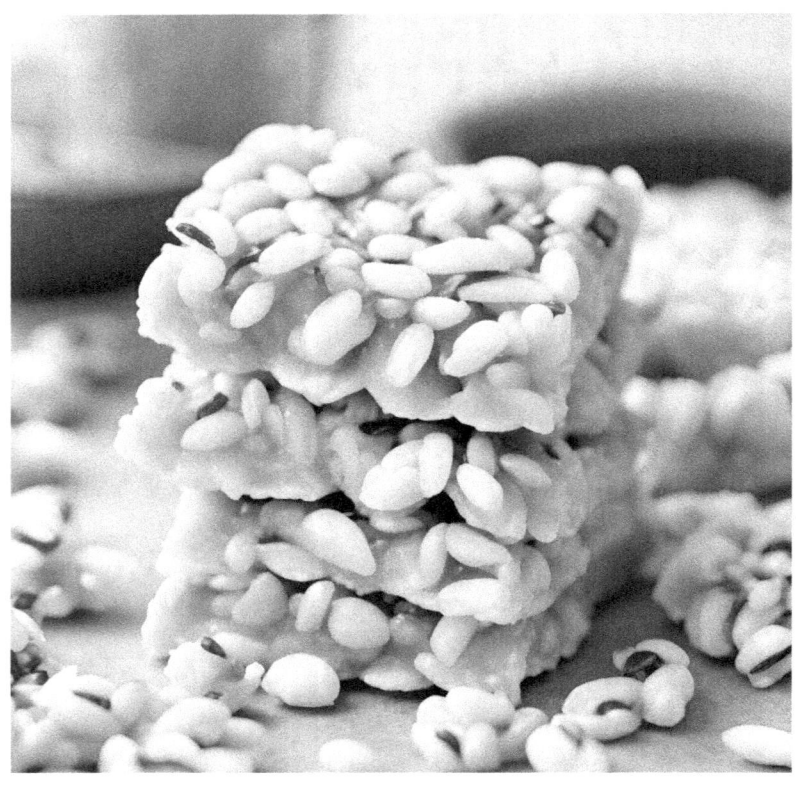

10. Lemon Pepper Cucumbers

Ingredients:
- 2 large cucumbers, thinly sliced
- 2 tablespoons olive oil
- 1 tablespoon lemon juice
- 1 teaspoon cracked black pepper

Instructions:
1. In a large bowl, combine sliced cucumbers, olive oil, lemon juice, and cracked black pepper.
2. Toss to coat the cucumbers evenly.
3. Chill in the refrigerator for about 30 minutes before serving to enhance the flavors.

Nutrition Info Per Serving:
- Calories: 80
- Protein: 1 g
- Carbohydrates: 4 g
- Fat: 7 g
- Sodium: 5 mg
- Potassium: 180 mg
- Phosphorus: 25 mg

Serves: 4 **Preparation Time:** 35 minutes

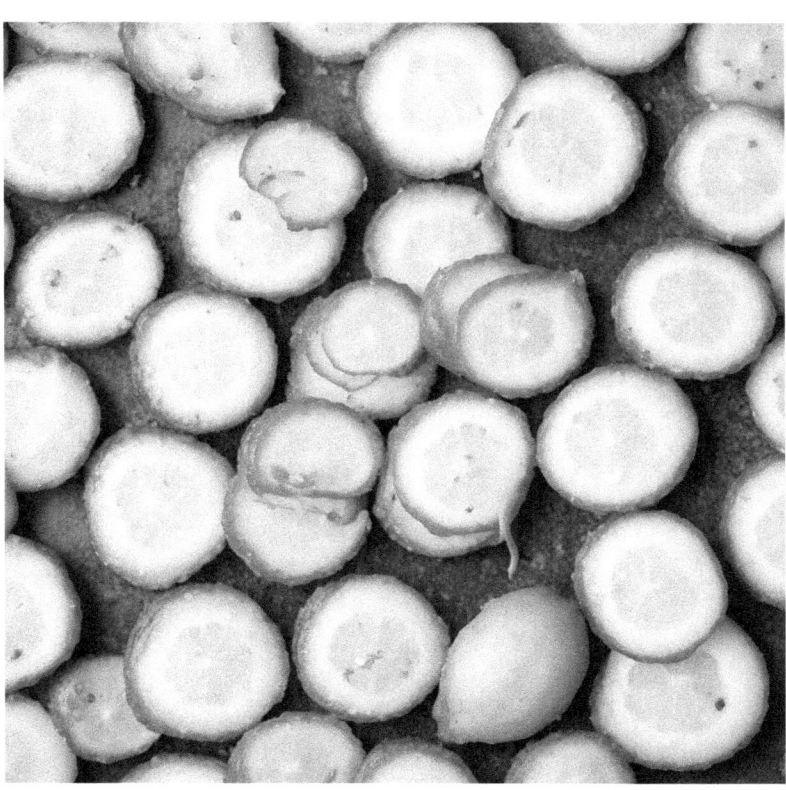

11. Pickled Radishes

Ingredients:
- 1 bunch radishes, thinly sliced
- 1 cup white vinegar
- 1 tablespoon sugar
- 1 clove garlic, minced
- 1 teaspoon mustard seeds

Instructions:
1. Place the sliced radishes in a jar.
2. In a saucepan, combine white vinegar, sugar, garlic, and mustard seeds. Bring to a boil.
3. Pour the boiling vinegar mixture over the radishes in the jar.
4. Let cool to room temperature, then seal and refrigerate.
5. Chill for at least 24 hours before serving.

Nutrition Info Per Serving:
- Calories: 25
- Protein: 1 g
- Carbohydrates: 4 g
- Fat: 0 g
- Sodium: 10 mg
- Potassium: 135 mg
- Phosphorus: 15 mg

Serves: 4 **Preparation Time:** 1 day

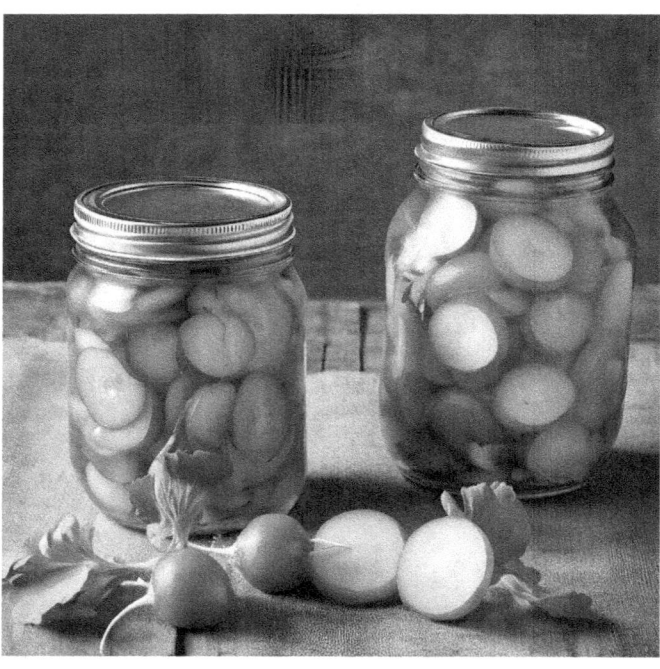

12. Steamed Carrots with Dill

Ingredients:
- 4 large carrots, peeled and sliced
- 2 tablespoons fresh dill, chopped
- 1 tablespoon olive oil

Instructions:
1. Steam carrots until they are tender, about 10-15 minutes.
2. Toss steamed carrots with olive oil and fresh dill.
3. Serve immediately.

Nutrition Info Per Serving:
- Calories: 80
- Protein: 1 g
- Carbohydrates: 10 g
- Fat: 4.5 g
- Sodium: 45 mg
- Potassium: 360 mg
- Phosphorus: 35 mg

Serves: 4 **Cooking Time:** 15 minutes

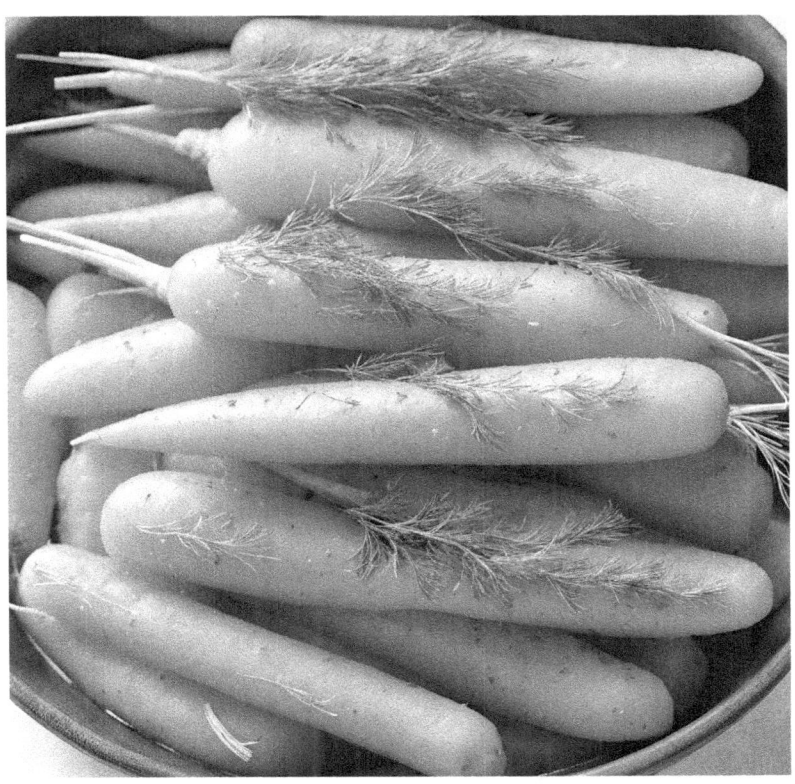

13. Mashed Turnips with Garlic

Ingredients:
- 4 large turnips, peeled and cubed
- 2 cloves garlic, minced
- 2 tablespoons olive oil
- 1/4 cup low-fat milk

Instructions:
1. Boil turnips until tender, about 20-25 minutes.
2. Drain and return turnips to the pot.
3. Add minced garlic, olive oil, and milk.
4. Mash until smooth.
5. Serve warm.

Nutrition Info Per Serving:
- Calories: 140
- Protein: 2 g
- Carbohydrates: 18 g
- Fat: 7 g
- Sodium: 50 mg
- Potassium: 280 mg
- Phosphorus: 60 mg

Serves: 4 **Cooking Time:** 30 minutes

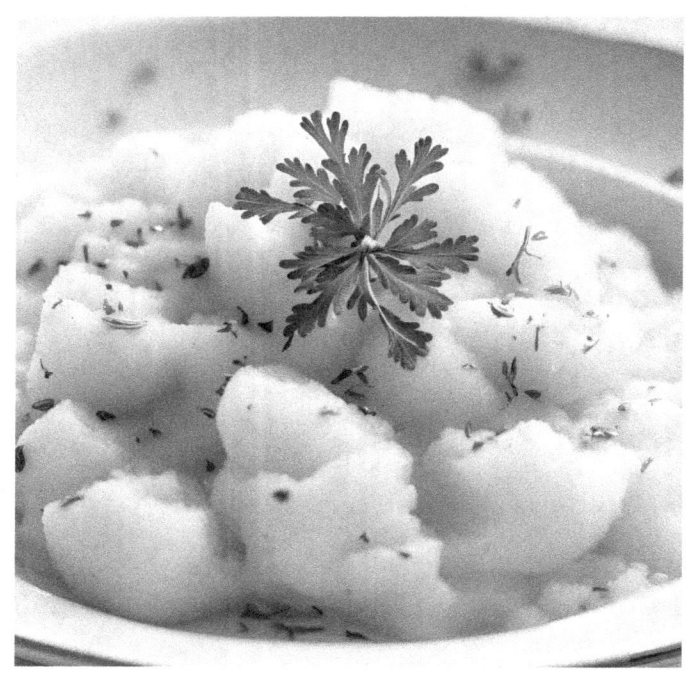

14. Sautéed Spinach with Garlic

Ingredients:
- 1 pound fresh spinach, washed
- 2 cloves garlic, minced
- 2 tablespoons olive oil

Instructions:
1. Heat olive oil in a large skillet over medium heat.
2. Add garlic and sauté for about 1 minute until fragrant.
3. Add spinach and cook until wilted, about 3-4 minutes.
4. Serve immediately.

Nutrition Info Per Serving:
- Calories: 90
- Protein: 3 g
- Carbohydrates: 4 g
- Fat: 7 g
- Sodium: 70 mg
- Potassium: 540 mg
- Phosphorus: 50 mg

Serves: 4 **Cooking Time:** 10 minutes

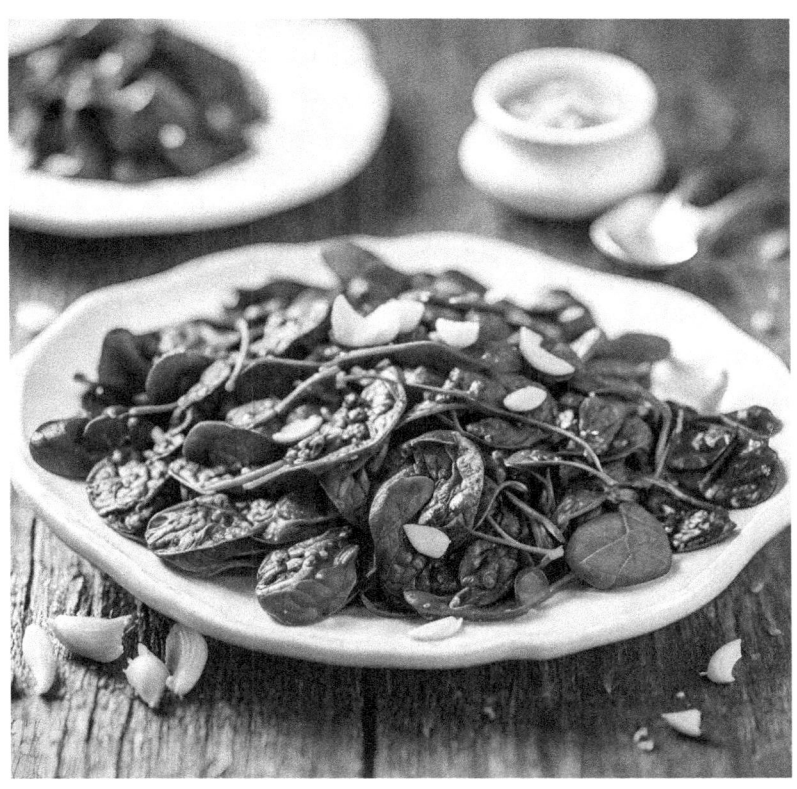

15. Onion and Herb Stuffed Mushrooms

Ingredients:
- 12 large button mushrooms, stems removed
- 1 onion, finely chopped
- 2 cloves garlic, minced
- 1/4 cup chopped fresh parsley
- 1/4 cup chopped fresh thyme
- 2 tablespoons olive oil
- 1/4 cup breadcrumbs

Instructions:
1. Preheat the oven to 375°F (190°C).
2. Heat one tablespoon of olive oil in a skillet over medium heat. Sauté onion and garlic until translucent.
3. In a bowl, mix sautéed onion and garlic with breadcrumbs, parsley, and thyme.
4. Stuff each mushroom cap with the mixture.
5. Place stuffed mushrooms on a baking sheet and drizzle with the remaining olive oil.
6. Bake for 20 minutes, or until the mushrooms are tender.
7. Serve warm.

Nutrition Info Per Serving:
- Calories: 60
- Protein: 2 g
- Carbohydrates: 6 g
- Fat: 3 g
- Sodium: 30 mg
- Potassium: 230 mg
- Phosphorus: 50 mg

Serves: 4 **Cooking Time:** 30 minutes

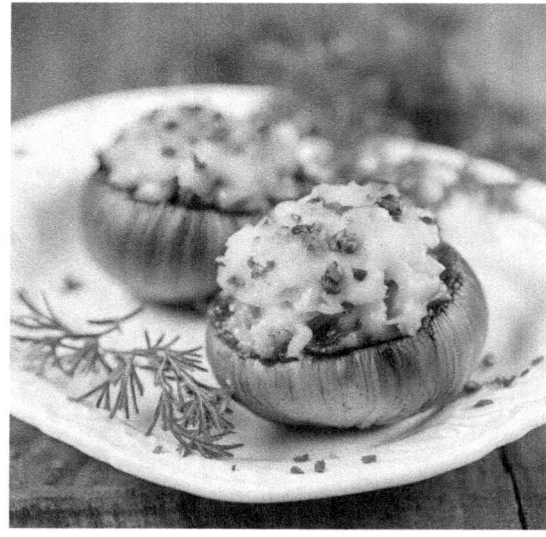

16. Roasted Beetroot

Ingredients:
- 4 medium beetroots, peeled and quartered
- 2 tablespoons olive oil
- 1 tablespoon balsamic vinegar

Instructions:
1. Preheat the oven to 400°F (200°C).
2. Toss beetroot quarters with olive oil and balsamic vinegar.
3. Place on a baking sheet and roast for 35-40 minutes, turning halfway through, until tender and caramelized.
4. Serve warm or at room temperature.

Nutrition Info Per Serving:
- Calories: 110
- Protein: 2 g
- Carbohydrates: 15 g
- Fat: 5 g
- Sodium: 65 mg
- Potassium: 450 mg
- Phosphorus: 40 mg

Serves: 4 **Cooking Time:** 40 minutes

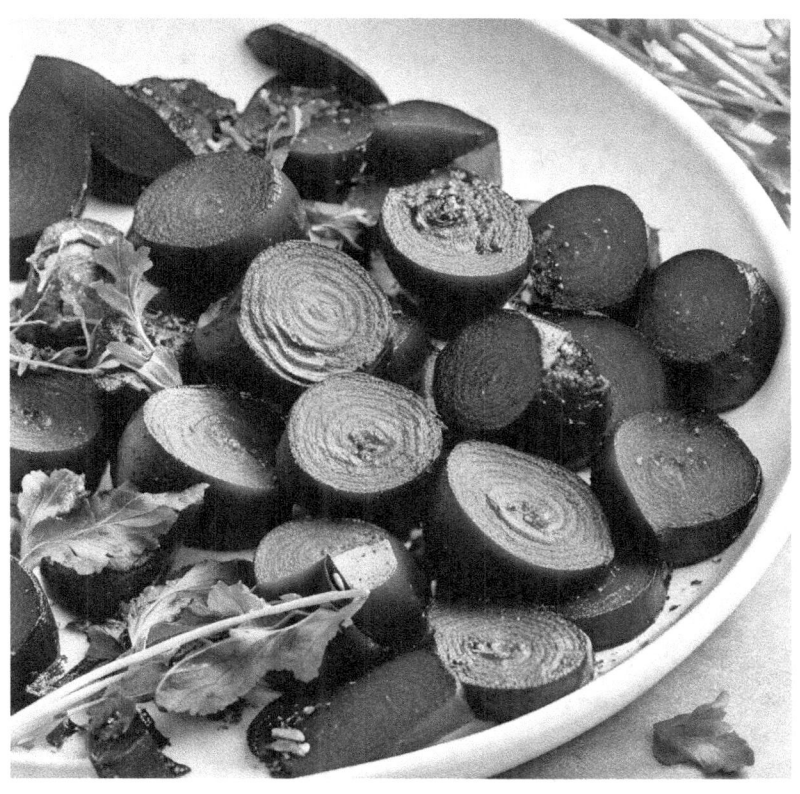

17. Green Bean Almondine

Ingredients:
- 1 pound green beans, trimmed
- 1/4 cup sliced almonds
- 2 tablespoons olive oil
- 1 tablespoon lemon juice

Instructions:
1. Steam green beans until tender-crisp, about 4-5 minutes.
2. Meanwhile, heat olive oil in a skillet over medium heat. Add almonds and toast until golden.
3. Add steamed green beans to the skillet, tossing with almonds and lemon juice.
4. Serve immediately.

Nutrition Info Per Serving:
- Calories: 150
- Protein: 4 g
- Carbohydrates: 8 g
- Fat: 12 g
- Sodium: 30 mg
- Potassium: 250 mg
- Phosphorus: 70 mg

Serves: 4 **Cooking Time:** 15 minutes

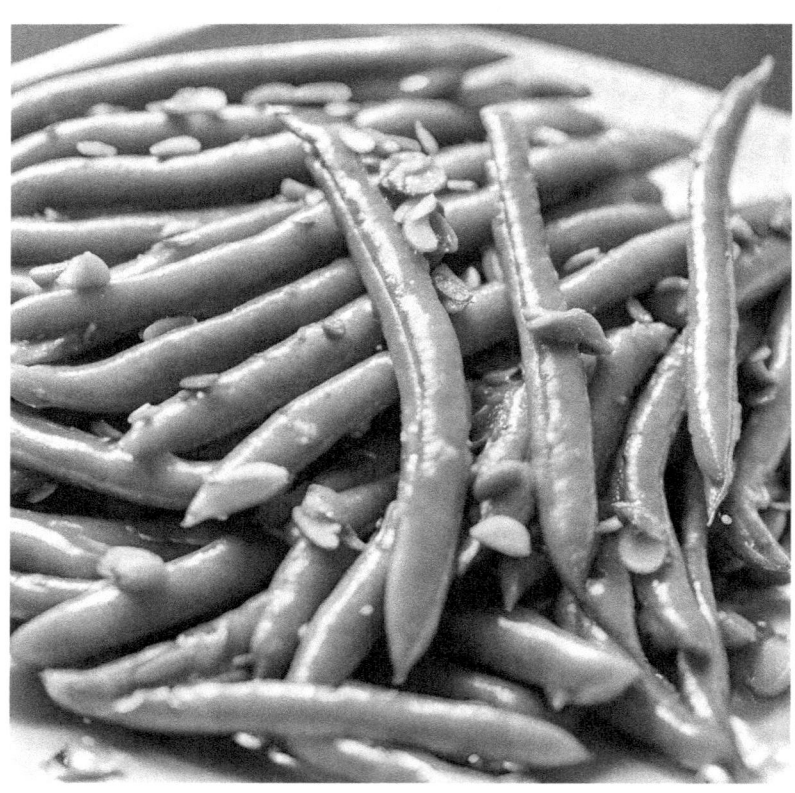

18. Pea and Carrot Salad

Ingredients:
- 1 cup peas (fresh or frozen, thawed)
- 1 cup carrots, diced and blanched
- 2 tablespoons olive oil
- 1 tablespoon apple cider vinegar
- 1 tablespoon fresh mint, chopped

Instructions:
1. In a salad bowl, combine peas and carrots.
2. In a small bowl, whisk together olive oil, apple cider vinegar, and chopped mint.
3. Pour the dressing over the peas and carrots and toss to coat.
4. Chill in the refrigerator for at least 30 minutes before serving.

Nutrition Info Per Serving:
- Calories: 130
- Protein: 2 g
- Carbohydrates: 10 g
- Fat: 9 g
- Sodium: 35 mg
- Potassium: 240 mg
- Phosphorus: 50 mg

Serves: 4 **Preparation Time:** 40 minutes

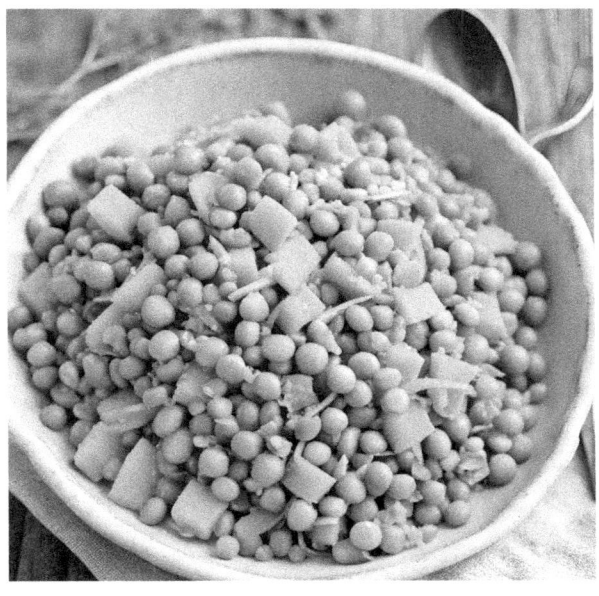

19. Oven-Roasted Leeks

Ingredients:
- 4 large leeks, cleaned and cut into 2-inch pieces
- 2 tablespoons olive oil
- 1 tablespoon lemon juice

Instructions:
1. Preheat the oven to 375°F (190°C).
2. Arrange the leek pieces in a single layer on a baking sheet.
3. Drizzle with olive oil and lemon juice.
4. Roast in the preheated oven for 25-30 minutes, or until the leeks are tender and beginning to caramelize at the edges.
5. Serve warm.

Nutrition Info Per Serving:
- Calories: 100
- Protein: 1 g
- Carbohydrates: 12 g
- Fat: 6 g
- Sodium: 20 mg
- Potassium: 160 mg
- Phosphorus: 35 mg

Serves: 4 **Cooking Time:** 30 minutes

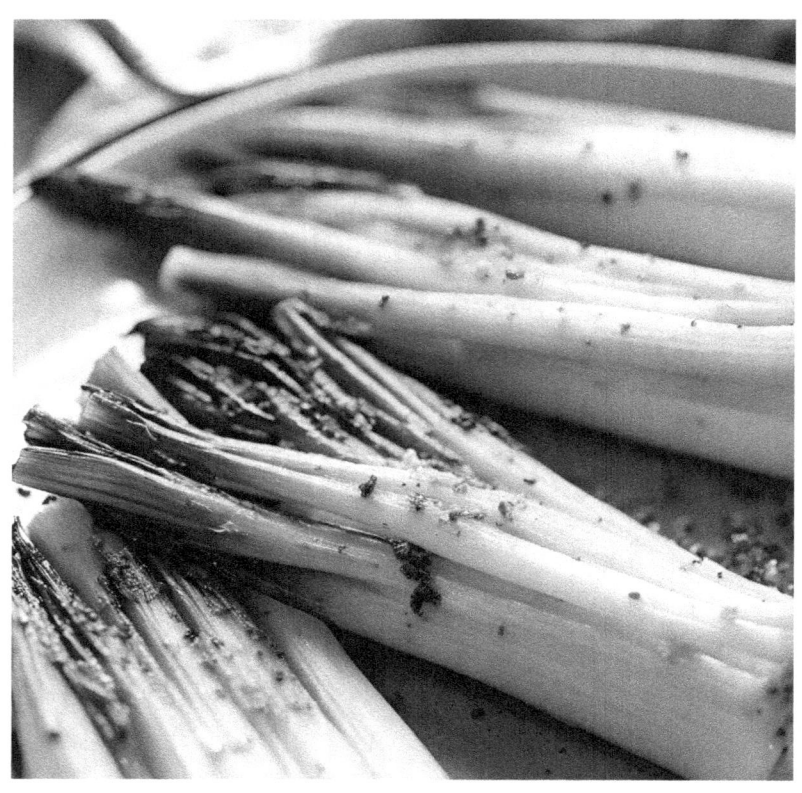

20. Chilled Cucumber Soup

Ingredients:
- 2 large cucumbers, peeled and chopped
- 1 cup plain low-fat yogurt
- 1 clove garlic, minced
- 1 tablespoon fresh dill, chopped
- 1 tablespoon lemon juice
- 1/4 cup cold water

Instructions:
1. In a blender, combine cucumbers, yogurt, garlic, dill, lemon juice, and water.
2. Blend until smooth.
3. Chill the soup in the refrigerator for at least 2 hours before serving.
4. Stir well before serving and adjust seasoning if necessary.

Nutrition Info Per Serving:
- Calories: 70
- Protein: 4 g
- Carbohydrates: 10 g
- Fat: 2 g
- Sodium: 30 mg
- Potassium: 250 mg
- Phosphorus: 45 mg

Serves: 4 **Preparation Time:** 10 minutes (plus at least 2 hours chilling)

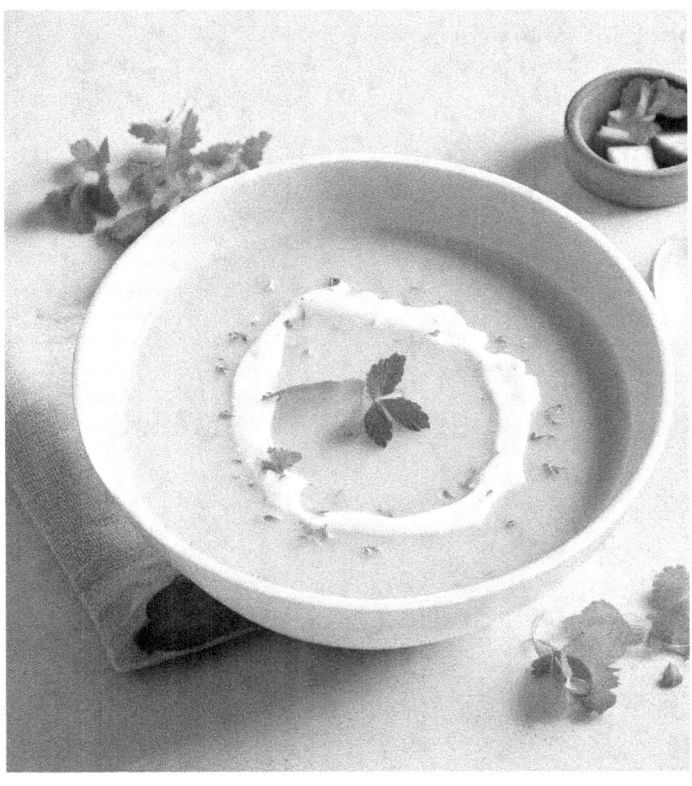

8-WEEK MEAL PLAN

Week 1

Day 1:
- **Breakfast:** Apple and Cinnamon Oatmeal
- **Lunch:** Cucumber Sandwiches
- **Dinner:** Garlic Butter Baked Tilapia with Steamed Carrots with Dill
- **Snack:** Apple Chips

Day 2:
- **Breakfast:** Blueberry Muffins
- **Lunch:** Summer Rice Salad
- **Dinner:** Vegetable Stir-Fry
- **Snack:** Rice Cakes with Unsweetened Apple Sauce

Day 3:
- **Breakfast:** Rice Pudding
- **Lunch:** Pasta Salad
- **Dinner:** Borscht (Beet Soup)
- **Snack:** Homemade Popcorn

Day 4:
- **Breakfast:** Peachy Keen Smoothie
- **Lunch:** Egg White Scramble
- **Dinner:** Lemon Herb Pasta
- **Snack:** Cucumber and Dill Bites

Day 5:
- **Breakfast:** Toast with Apple Butter
- **Lunch:** Roasted Bell Pepper Soup
- **Dinner:** Sautéed Mushrooms and Onions with Mashed Turnips with Garlic
- **Snack:** Garlic Toast

Day 6:
- **Breakfast:** Cream of Wheat
- **Lunch:** Rice Paper Rolls
- **Dinner:** Roasted Beetroot with Green Bean Almondine
- **Snack:** Zucchini Chips

Day 7:
- **Breakfast:** Vegetable Hash
- **Lunch:** Egg Salad
- **Dinner:** Onion and Herb Stuffed Mushrooms with a side of Mixed Greens with Apple Slices
- **Snack:** Puffed Rice Bars

Week 2

Day 8:
- **Breakfast:** Polenta Porridge
- **Lunch:** Celery Sticks with Hummus
- **Dinner:** Baked Parsnip Fries with Herb-Roasted Potatoes
- **Snack:** Lemon Pepper Cucumbers

Day 9:
- **Breakfast:** Cranberry Scones
- **Lunch:** Carrot Ginger Soup
- **Dinner:** Cucumber Gazpacho
- **Snack:** Pickled Radishes

Day 10:
- **Breakfast:** Pineapple Rice Breakfast Bowl
- **Lunch:** Cauliflower Steak
- **Dinner:** Parsley and Lemon Pasta
- **Snack:** Steamed Carrots with Dill

Day 11:
- **Breakfast:** Stuffed Avocado
- **Lunch:** Mixed Berry Salad
- **Dinner:** Asparagus Soup
- **Snack:** Carrot Sticks with Homemade Tzatziki

Day 12:
- **Breakfast:** Cherry Almond Bars
- **Lunch:** Garlic Mashed Potatoes
- **Dinner:** Squash and Apple Soup
- **Snack:** Endive and Pear Salad

Day 13:
- **Breakfast:** Pearled Barley with Apples
- **Lunch:** Vegetable Kabobs
- **Dinner:** Iceberg Lettuce with Radishes
- **Snack:** Jicama Salad

Day 14:
- **Breakfast:** Zucchini Bread
- **Lunch:** Cornmeal Porridge
- **Dinner:** Shredded Beet and Carrot Salad
- **Snack:** Oven-Roasted Leeks

Week 3

Day 15:
- **Breakfast:** Oat Bran Muffins
- **Lunch:** Pumpkin Soup
- **Dinner:** Radish and Green Onion Salad
- **Snack:** Chilled Cucumber Soup

Day 16:
- **Breakfast:** Maple Syrup Granola
- **Lunch:** Lemon Ricotta Pancakes
- **Dinner:** Pea and Carrot Salad
- **Snack:** Apple Chips

Day 17:
- **Breakfast:** Buckwheat Porridge
- **Lunch:** Strawberry Smoothie
- **Dinner:** Celery Soup
- **Snack:** Rice Cakes with Unsweetened Apple Sauce

Day 18:
- **Breakfast:** Barley Vegetable Soup
- **Lunch:** Leek and Potato Soup
- **Dinner:** Green Bean Soup
- **Snack:** Homemade Popcorn

Day 19:
- **Breakfast:** Turnip Soup
- **Lunch:** Asparagus Soup
- **Dinner:** Squash and Apple Soup
- **Snack:**

Cucumber and Dill Bites

Day 20:
- **Breakfast:** Cucumber Dill Soup
- **Lunch:** Parsnip Soup
- **Dinner:** Red Bell Pepper Soup
- **Snack:** Garlic Toast

Day 21:
- **Breakfast:** Puffed Rice Bars
- **Lunch:** Baked Parsnip Fries
- **Dinner:** Zucchini Chips
- **Snack:** Lemon Pepper Cucumbers

Week 4

Day 1:
- **Breakfast:** Cornflake cereal with Almond Milk
- **Lunch:** Borscht (Beet Soup)
- **Dinner:** Garlic Spinach Sauté with Grilled Zucchini and Squash
- **Snack:** Apple Chips

Day 2:
- **Breakfast:** Lemon Herb Pasta
- **Lunch:** Cucumber Sandwiches
- **Dinner:** Roasted Root Vegetables
- **Snack:** Carrot Sticks with Homemade Tzatziki

Day 3:
- **Breakfast:** Vegetable Hash
- **Lunch:** Egg Salad
- **Dinner:** Chilled Asparagus Salad
- **Snack:** Zucchini Chips

Day 4:
- **Breakfast:** Buckwheat Porridge
- **Lunch:** Parsley and Lemon Pasta
- **Dinner:** Roasted Bell Pepper Salad
- **Snack:** Homemade Popcorn

Day 5:
- **Breakfast:** Cream of Wheat
- **Lunch:** Pasta Salad
- **Dinner:** Onion and Herb Stuffed Mushrooms
- **Snack:** Rice Cakes with Unsweetened Apple Sauce

Day 6:
- **Breakfast:** Rice Pudding
- **Lunch:** Leek and Potato Soup
- **Dinner:** Endive and Pear Salad
- **Snack:** Puffed Rice Bars

Day 7:
- **Breakfast:** Cranberry Scones
- **Lunch:** Green Bean Soup
- **Dinner:** Lemon Pepper Cucumbers
- **Snack:** Cucumber and Dill Bites

Week 5

Day 8:
- **Breakfast:** Peachy Keen Smoothie
- **Lunch:** Summer Rice Salad
- **Dinner:** Tomato and Cucumber Gazpacho Salad
- **Snack:** Garlic Toast

Day 9:
- **Breakfast:** Pearled Barley with Apples
- **Lunch:** Turnip Soup
- **Dinner:** Pickled Radishes
- **Snack:** Apple Chips

Day 10:
- **Breakfast:** Mixed Berry Salad
- **Lunch:** Rice Paper Rolls
- **Dinner:** Jicama Salad
- **Snack:** Carrot Sticks with Homemade Tzatziki

Day 11:
- **Breakfast:** Zucchini Bread
- **Lunch:** Celery Soup
- **Dinner:** Squash and Apple Soup
- **Snack:** Zucchini Chips

Day 12:
- **Breakfast:** Oat Bran Muffins
- **Lunch:** Tomato and Basil Bruschetta
- **Dinner:** Radish and Green Onion Salad
- **Snack:** Homemade Popcorn

Day 13:
- **Breakfast:** Blueberry Muffins
- **Lunch:** Carrot Ginger Soup
- **Dinner:** Shredded Beet and Carrot Salad
- **Snack:** Rice Cakes with Unsweetened Apple Sauce

Day 14:
- **Breakfast:** Toast with Apple Butter
- **Lunch:** Mixed Vegetable Grill
- **Dinner:** Oven-Roasted Leeks
- **Snack:** Puffed Rice Bars

Week 6

Day 15:
- **Breakfast:** Polenta Porridge
- **Lunch:** Cabbage Stir-Fry
- **Dinner:** Iceberg Lettuce with Radishes
- **Snack:** Apple Chips

Day 16:
- **Breakfast:** Cherry Almond Bars
- **Lunch:** Asparagus Soup
- **Dinner:** Pea and Carrot Salad
- **Snack:** Carrot Sticks with Homemade Tzatziki

Day 17:
- **Breakfast:** Pearled Barley with Apples
- **Lunch:** Cucumber Gazpacho
- **Dinner:** Chilled Cucumber Soup
- **Snack:** Zucchini Chips

Day 18:
- **Breakfast:** Vegetable Hash
- **Lunch:** Roasted Beetroot
- **Dinner:** Green Bean Almondine
- **Snack:** Homemade Popcorn

Day 19:
- **Breakfast:** Rice Pudding
- **Lunch:** Lemon Ricotta Pancakes
- **Dinner:** Steamed Carrots with Dill
- **Snack:** Rice Cakes with Unsweetened Apple Sauce

Day 20:
- **Breakfast:** Maple Syrup Granola
- **Lunch:** Egg White Scramble
- **Dinner:** Mixed Greens with Apple Slices
- **Snack:** Puffed Rice Bars

Day 21:
- **Breakfast:** Buckwheat Porridge
- **Lunch:** Stuffed Tomato with Rice
- **Dinner:** Mashed Turnips with Garlic
- **Snack:** Cucumber and Dill Bites

Week 7

Day 22:
- **Breakfast:** Cornflake cereal with Almond Milk
- **Lunch:** Strawberry Smoothie
- **Dinner:** Sautéed Spinach with Garlic
- **Snack:** Garlic Toast

Day 23:
- **Breakfast:** Lemon Herb Pasta
- **Lunch:** Iceberg Lettuce with Radishes
- **Dinner:** Roasted Root Vegetables
- **Snack:** Apple Chips

Day 24:
- **Breakfast:** Cherry Almond Bars
- **Lunch:** Endive and Pear Salad
- **Dinner:** Onion and Herb Stuffed Mushrooms
- **Snack:** Zucchini Chips

Day 25:
- **Breakfast:** Vegetable Hash
- **Lunch:** Baked Parsnip Fries
- **Dinner:** Lemon Pepper Cucumbers
- **Snack:** Carrot Sticks with Homemade Tzatziki

Day 26:
- **Breakfast:** Buckwheat Porridge
- **Lunch:** Parsley and Lemon Pasta
- **Dinner:** Pickled Radishes
- **Snack:** Homemade Popcorn

Day 27:
- **Breakfast:** Rice Pudding
- **Lunch:** Steamed Carrots with Dill
- **Dinner:** Jicama Salad
- **Snack:** Rice Cakes with Unsweetened Apple Sauce

Day 28:
- **Breakfast:** Toast with Apple Butter
- **Lunch:** Tomato and Basil Bruschetta
- **Dinner:** Radish and Green Onion Salad
- **Snack:** Puffed Rice Bars

Week 8

Day 29:
- **Breakfast:** Polenta Porridge
- **Lunch:** Summer Rice Salad
- **Dinner:** Squash and Apple Soup
- **Snack:** Garlic Toast

Day 30:
- **Breakfast:** Blueberry Muffins
- **Lunch:** Egg Salad
- **Dinner:** Shredded Beet and Carrot Salad
- **Snack:** Apple Chips

Day 31:
- **Breakfast:** Cream of Wheat
- **Lunch:** Mixed Vegetable Grill
- **Dinner:** Oven-Roasted Leeks
- **Snack:** Zucchini Chips

Day 32:
- **Breakfast:** Cranberry Scones
- **Lunch:** Cabbage Stir-Fry
- **Dinner:** Pea and Carrot Salad
- **Snack:** Carrot Sticks with Homemade Tzatziki

Day 33:
- **Breakfast:** Peachy Keen Smoothie
- **Lunch:** Leek and Potato Soup
- **Dinner:** Green Bean Almondine
- **Snack:** Homemade Popcorn

Day 34:
- **Breakfast:** Pearled Barley with Apples
- **Lunch:** Turnip Soup
- **Dinner:** Iceberg Lettuce with Radishes
- **Snack:** Rice Cakes with Unsweetened Apple Sauce

Day 35:
- **Breakfast:** Zucchini Bread
- **Lunch:** Celery Soup
- **Dinner:** Chilled Cucumber Soup
- **Snack:** Puffed Rice Bars

MEAL PLANNER JOURNAL

	BREAKFAST	LUNCH	DINNER	SNACKS
MON				
TUE				
WED				
THU				
FRI				
SAT				
SUN				

What are your primary symptoms of kidney disease, and how do they impact your everyday life?

MEAL PLANNER JOURNAL

	BREAKFAST	LUNCH	DINNER	SNACKS
MON				
TUE				
WED				
THU				
FRI				
SAT				
SUN				

What are your top three goals for starting the kidney disease diet?

MEAL PLANNER JOURNAL

	BREAKFAST	LUNCH	DINNER	SNACKS
MON				
TUE				
WED				
THU				
FRI				
SAT				
SUN				

Which foods do you currently enjoy that might need to be limited or avoided on the kidney disease diet?

MEAL PLANNER JOURNAL

	BREAKFAST	LUNCH	DINNER	SNACKS
MON				
TUE				
WED				
THU				
FRI				
SAT				
SUN				

How do you feel about making significant dietary changes to manage your kidney disease?

MEAL PLANNER JOURNAL

	BREAKFAST	LUNCH	DINNER	SNACKS
MON				
TUE				
WED				
THU				
FRI				
SAT				
SUN				

Describe a typical day's meals and snacks before beginning the kidney disease diet.

MEAL PLANNER JOURNAL

	BREAKFAST	LUNCH	DINNER	SNACKS
MON				
TUE				
WED				
THU				
FRI				
SAT				
SUN				

What challenges or concerns do you anticipate facing while following the kidney disease diet?

MEAL PLANNER JOURNAL

	BREAKFAST	LUNCH	DINNER	SNACKS
MON				
TUE				
WED				
THU				
FRI				
SAT				
SUN				

List three kidney-friendly foods you are looking forward to incorporating into your meals.

MEAL PLANNER JOURNAL

	BREAKFAST	LUNCH	DINNER	SNACKS
MON				
TUE				
WED				
THU				
FRI				
SAT				
SUN				

How do you plan to navigate dining out or attending social gatherings while adhering to the kidney disease diet?

MEAL PLANNER JOURNAL

	BREAKFAST	LUNCH	DINNER	SNACKS
MON				
TUE				
WED				
THU				
FRI				
SAT				
SUN				

What new recipes or cooking methods are you excited to try on the kidney disease diet?

MEAL PLANNER JOURNAL

	BREAKFAST	LUNCH	DINNER	SNACKS
MON				
TUE				
WED				
THU				
FRI				
SAT				
SUN				

Reflect on any previous attempts to manage your kidney disease through diet. What were the successes and challenges?

MEAL PLANNER JOURNAL

	BREAKFAST	LUNCH	DINNER	SNACKS
MON				
TUE				
WED				
THU				
FRI				
SAT				
SUN				

What strategies will you use to stay motivated and committed to the kidney disease diet during difficult times?

MEAL PLANNER JOURNAL

	BREAKFAST	LUNCH	DINNER	SNACKS
MON				
TUE				
WED				
THU				
FRI				
SAT				
SUN				

Who are your support systems (friends, family, healthcare providers) that can help you with your dietary changes?

MEAL PLANNER JOURNAL

	BREAKFAST	LUNCH	DINNER	SNACKS
MON				
TUE				
WED				
THU				
FRI				
SAT				
SUN				

How do you anticipate your quality of life improving by following the kidney disease diet?

Scan the QR code below to get a surprise bonus!

www.ingramcontent.com/pod-product-compliance
Lightning Source LLC
Chambersburg PA
CBHW082206220526
45470CB00010B/3059